THE
GYM-FREE
JOURNAL

Bodyweight Workouts for Getting Ripped

Brett Stewart

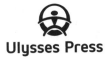

Ulysses Press

Published in the United States by
Ulysses Press
P.O. Box 3440
Berkeley, CA 94703
www.ulyssespress.com

ISBN13: 978-1-61243-277-9
Library of Congress Control Number 2013947495

Printed in the United States by United Graphics Inc.

10 9 8 7 6 5 4 3 2 1

Acquisitions Editor: Katherine Furman
Managing Editor: Claire Chun
Editor: Lauren Harrison
Proofreader: Lily Chou
Index: Sayre Van Young
Cover design: what!design@whatweb.com
Interior design: Jake Flaherty
Cover photographs: woman © Maksim Shmeljov/shutterstock.com; man © Standret/
    shutterstock.com
Models: Evan Clontz, Lewis Elliot, Brett Stewart
Interior photographs: © Rapt Productions except page 5 © hobbit/shutterstock.com; page 27 ©
    Enigmangels/shutterstock.com; page 213 © Maffi/shutterstock.com

Distributed by Publishers Group West

PLEASE NOTE: This book has been written and published strictly for informational purposes, and in no way should be used as a substitute for consultation with health care professionals. You should not consider educational material herein to be the practice of medicine or to replace consultation with a physician or other medical practitioner. The author and publisher are providing you with information in this work so that you can have the knowledge and can choose, at your own risk, to act on that knowledge. The author and publisher also urge all readers to be aware of their health status and to consult health care professionals before beginning any health program.

CONTENTS

PART 1: OVERVIEW

INTRODUCTION

So, you want to get ripped (or shredded, jacked, buff, toned, built, cut and any number of cute little terms to depict a chiseled, Adonis-like physique)? Well, maybe not. How about losing weight, getting healthier and being fit? How about FIT, or Function in Training—where you'll use a myriad of bodyweight exercises that simulate real-world (functional) movements to strengthen, shape and tone your entire body. These functional movements are simple to learn, remember and replicate from day to day and workout to workout. The goal of *The Gym-Free Journal* is very simple: We'll use FIT to get you fit!

Let's say your goal is to get in shape—really in shape—and develop the physique that guys and gals alike want to attain. How do you do it? Where do you start? If you watch any commercial for weight-loss pills or crazy fitness contraptions, you'll see some dude with six-pack abs, bulging arms and a chiseled chest posing next to a babe with amazing legs, a flat tummy and all the right assets. They smile at the camera and tell you that it's fast, fun and easy to get ripped in just weeks with some incredible diet pill or the BellyRipper2000. You know they're pulling your leg, right? Usually, these models have never even seen the product they're pitching before the video shoot.

So, who do you believe? Should you trust the companies that spend hundreds of thousands of dollars on infomercials? Should you put all your faith in a miracle fat-burning pill? Are you only going to get results if you pay hundreds of dollars a month to a personal trainer? You know the real answer—it's been there all along and is even easier than you think. Trust your body. Get active, eat healthily and get ripped—that's it.

To most people, building a workout routine is a mystery. Should you do heavy weights and low reps or light weights and high reps? Should you work in supersets or target muscles? Upper body or lower body? Kettlebells, sprints, squats, stairs, pyramids, yadda yadda yadda?

There are more ways to work out than you can count, and they all have their benefits. If you pick up any fitness magazine you'll learn about different "must do" exercises that sometimes conflict with other routines in that same issue! How on earth can you make sense of the information overload and develop an efficient way to get the ripped results you want? Since you're reading this, you no longer have to.

Here's some good news: You can get in the best shape of your life more quickly than you ever thought possible by following a simple program of easy-to-do bodyweight exercises and equally simple nutritional guidelines. The even better news is that you don't need any expensive gadgets, a gym membership or even a personal trainer. You're holding in your hands a book devoted to taking the mystery out of getting ripped and showing you step by step how to attain the body you want. With easy-to-follow and simple-to-remember programs that average 20 minutes a day, you can seamlessly adapt to a fit lifestyle and reap all the benefits of being in shape: playing with your kids, beating your older brother at hoops, conquering a Spartan Race or even enjoying the pursuit of fitness itself—a walk, jog or activity that you can do all by yourself or with friends of family.

The act of getting fit is only a chore if you make it one. Getting and staying in shape can actually be fun if you make it so, and it starts with a positive mental attitude. If you find yourself saying, "Ugh, I need to go do my work out," then you're not going to stick with it. By adding some fun activities to your daily routine along with just a little positive thinking, you should be able to turn that into, "Yes, I get to take one more step on my fitness journey today!" Still have doubts? Well, this is your option to prove to yourself that you can and will succeed in your fitness goals!

Your Roadmap

I have one of the best "jobs" in the world: I write books about fitness and train with some of the coolest professional, amateur and beginner athletes in the world. My books have taken me to some amazing places all over the United States, from racing a Spartan Race in the middle of the Arizona desert to running a marathon in the mountains of Montana. I've spent countless hours with professional triathletes, runners and obstacle racers to get the inside scoop on training, nutrition and motivation to compete at the highest levels.

Without question, the most rewarding experiences I've had come from working with beginners. Whether they're first-timers running in a 5K, triathlon, marathon or mud run, these athletes are always the most fun to work with, teach and learn from as they progress through their fitness journeys. Why? Well, all the energy in the form of excitement and nerves that they bring to each workout, for one thing. Each new step on their expedition from out-of-shape individual to fit athlete (and yes, that's a relative term) is met with initial trepidation and eventually completed with a resounding "aha!" when they realize that they have the ability and drive to reach their goals. Newbies (beginners) have the most ground to gain on their quest, more distance to cover step by step to reach their goals. I personally love being along for the ride and am thrilled to provide this book as your roadmap to point you in the right direction, give you a little kick in the butt to get you going, and give as many tips as I can to keep you on track along the way.

Do you need a roadmap on your fitness journey? Absolutely. My favorite Yogi Berra quote is, "If you don't know where you're going, you may end up somewhere else." Well, fitness is the same way. Too often we all (me included!) develop "workout ADD" where we jump from one program to the next without taking the time to develop consistency and see results in a particular one first. While all exercise is good for your physique, deviating from a plan and just doing the exercises you feel like doing will yield marginal results. Even worse, doing the same exercises at the same weight on the same day will lead to plateaus where your body adapts to the stimulus (the workout) and stops getting stronger. Once you get to that stage, you're sufficiently bored and end up quitting exercise altogether instead of continuing with the same old, same old. Even if you do up the intensity of these exercises, you're still cruisin' for a bruisin' by potentially overtraining the same muscles, resulting in plateaus, burnouts and injury!

The programs in this book are designed for ease of use; you don't have to do any calculations or learn any complicated routines. Monday, Wednesday, and Friday you'll have a 20-minute workout to complete and then go on with your hectic day. Whether you're an early riser, a lunchtime exerciser, an afternoon gym-goer, or a late-night runner, you can surely find 20 minutes to help make you stronger, faster and fitter—right?

The rule of thumb for any lifestyle modification is that it takes anywhere from 7 to 14 days to create a new routine, and this book will make it as easy as possible to get started—and succeed. Your success depends on building a sustainable routine that's familiar, comfortable and repeatable. Working out is hard enough without having to get up early to drive to the gym, remember how to use complicated machines and figure out your daily workout (not to mention locating your membership card!). You can get an incredible full-body workout right in the comfort of your home, saving yourself precious time and gas by not traveling to the gym. You don't even need an expensive rack of dumbbells, bars or how-to DVDs—all you need is your body (you have one of those, right?), a pull-up bar, and maybe a ball or two.

Why Bodyweight Exercises?

This is a really simple answer: because they work. Your body is the only gym you should ever need. Sure, some gyms have amazing amenities—but you can't take 'em with you. Your body is a lot more portable than a Smith machine, isn't it? Through balance, stability and mobility, bodyweight exercises also strengthen you in ways that no gym equipment ever can. In order to be "fit," you need to be able to incorporate all the muscles in your body when you squat, twist, reach or jump in sports or everyday life. Strengthening your body by actually using your own bodyweight is natural and involves stimulating muscles through a normal range of motion. Lying flat on a bench or sitting while you pull a bar down is absolutely no match for the full-body strength gains and ripped physique you can get from doing bodyweight exercises with proper form. Most importantly, using your own bodyweight to get fit is simple, repeatable and always available. It's much easier to sneak in a few sets of bodyweight exercises than it is to pack up and drive to the gym! The more convenient a workout is, the more apt you are to complete it. Throw in some fun and your workouts are downright enjoyable. At the end of the day, the investment of time that you put into bodyweight exercises is so much less than a gym-based workout routine and it's actually more effective at developing total-body fitness. Oh, and better yet, it's free.

THE MUSCLES BEHIND THE MOVEMENTS

The programs in *The Gym-Free Journal* will work all major muscle groups and most ancillary muscles in your body, but instead of covering the function of all 640 muscles, we'll break the body down into two generic sections: "movers" and "core."

Movers are any muscle whose prime movement is to push, pull or rotate any part of your body aside from your core. The core is the foundation that allows the movers to do their thing and handles twisting and crunching. The stronger your core is, the more effective, efficient and enduring all your mover muscles will be. Building your core strength is the key to total-body fitness and absolutely imperative when developing a fit, ripped physique. Throughout the book, we'll focus on exercises that use at least one from each group. Most will use both, and at least one exercise will use all of the above. Seriously, it'll use all of them.

MOVERS

PECTORALIS MAJOR   This pair of thick, fan-shaped muscles makes up the bulk of the muscle mass in the chest. The "pecs" are responsible for rotating, flexing and bringing in both arms for actions such as throwing a ball, lifting a child, or performing jumping jacks or push-ups.

TRICEPS BRACHII   The large muscle located on the back of the upper arm, the triceps brachii (commonly referred to as "triceps") is responsible for straightening the arm. The triceps makes up over 50 percent of the upper arm's muscular mass.

DELTOID   This heart-shaped muscle group is made up of three different fibers (front, middle and rear). While each fiber type has a specific function, the "delts" as a whole are responsible for raising and stabilizing the arms during rotation.

BICEPS BRACHII   One of the assisting muscles during a pull-up, the biceps brachii (commonly referred to as "biceps") is responsible for forearm rotation and elbow flexion. It's located on the front of the upper arm. *Note:* Chin-ups are more effective at targeting the biceps than pull-ups are due to the supinated grip.

TRAPEZIUS   Another prime mover, the trapezius (commonly referred to as "traps") is a large, superficial muscle located between the base of the skull and the mid-back, and laterally between both shoulders. Its primary function is to move the scapulae (shoulder blades) and support the arm.

LATISSIMUS DORSI   The latissimus dorsi (meaning "broadest muscle in the back") is responsible for moving the arm toward the center of the body (adduction), internally rotating the arm at the shoulder toward the center of the body (medial rotation), and moving the arm straight back behind the body (posterior shoulder extension). It also plays a synergistic role in extending and bending to either side (lateral flexion) the lumbar spine. This pair of muscles is commonly referred to as the "lats."

FOREARM FLEXORS/EXTENSORS   The structure between the elbow and wrist contains a number of muscles, including the flexors and extensors of the digits, brachioradialis (which flexes the elbow), pronators (which turn the palm of the hand downward) and supinator (which turns the palm of the hand upward). These muscles allow you to grip the bar during a pull-up.

GLUTEUS MAXIMUS   This muscle makes up the majority of the buttocks and is responsible for maintaining an erect posture, raising from a squat position and performing most leg motions, such as adduction and rotation.

QUADRICEPS   The quadriceps is a large muscle group made up of four muscles on the front of the thigh. It's the strongest, leanest muscle mass on the body. The "quads" are responsible for straightening the knee joint and are crucial in walking, running, squatting and jumping.

HAMSTRINGS   The hamstrings, located on the back of the thigh, are made up of four muscles responsible for knee bending and hip straightening. The hamstrings work as antagonists to the quadriceps to enable walking, running and jumping, as well as maintaining stability in the hip and knee.

CALVES   The triceps surae, or "calves," is made up of the gastrocnemius and soleus muscles. These muscles attach to the Achilles tendon and are responsible for ankle rotation, flexion and stabilization, and are crucial for walking, running and jumping.

CORE

This term refers to the area of the torso composed of the rectus abdominis (the "six-pack" portion of the abdominals), obliques, transversus abdominis and erector spinae. Full-body functional movements traditionally originate from this area of the body, and it provides stabilization during pretty much every activity your body performs on a daily basis, from exercises including the pull-up to maintaining proper posture when standing or sitting. A strong core is essential to proper fitness; your body's strength needs a solid base to work from.

FREQUENTLY ASKED QUESTIONS

Q. Can't I just do crunches to rip my abs?

A. You can do crunches all day long and still not have a ripped core. Period. Unless you work your entire body to get lean, you just won't be able to show off your six-pack.

Q. I was always told to stretch first, but lately I've read that you shouldn't stretch your muscles when you're cold. What's the deal?

A. Research and studies over the last few years have reinforced the reasoning that you should warm up before you exercise and then stretch after you've completed your workout. Read more about warming up and stretching on page 231.

Q. Isn't it true that bodyweight exercises don't make your muscles as big as gym-based exercises?

A. If you want to build the biggest chest possible by loading up a bar and doing reps of bench press over and over, this is probably the wrong book for you. But remember, you can build huge arms, pecs and legs and still be unfit—unable to perform well at the complex motions necessary for most sports. Using bodyweight exercises, you'll build your entire body and the end result will be a stronger, faster and fitter version of you. You'll also be amazed at how much bigger muscles look when you're ripped.

Q. Can I do a full-body workout every day?

A. No, your body needs time to rest and recover. When you do strength-training exercises such as pull-ups, you create tiny, harmless tears in the muscle. These tiny tears heal during rest days. As a result, the muscle becomes stronger and more defined. If you don't allow the muscles to heal, you risk overuse injuries that could potentially derail your ability to exercise at all. Constant repetitions of any motion without proper rest will eventually result in overuse injuries. Repeat this sentence: "Rest is equally as important as the workout for strengthening and shredding your body." Now, make sure you follow your own advice.

Q. What if I can't do all the reps in the program for a given workout?

A. The reps are a guideline and a goal for each workout—they're not the law. I can promise you that no one will show up at your door to give you a ticket for missing the last two reps of pull-ups. Do as many reps as you can with good form and when you reach failure, your body is signaling that you're done. If you still feel like you have some fuel left in the tank, then take a break for 1–2 minutes and try to finish off the set. If you feel any pain, soreness or dizziness, then it's time to call it a day. Never feel ashamed that you didn't complete every rep of a workout—stay positive and come back strong after a day of rest.

If you missed more than 30 percent of the reps, I suggest starting over the same workout after you've rested and recovered. Feel free to progress onward if it's just one or two reps, but be honest with yourself if you find yourself missing reps every workout—perform the exercises within your ability and you'll get stronger and eventually be able to complete the full workout.

Q. How fast should I do the movements?

A. Some exercises will have specific speeds during certain workouts, but as a rule of thumb you should try to stick to a "medium" speed. Listen to your body; you'll know what's too fast or too slow with a little bit of experience. If you're just learning the movements, take it as slowly as you need to maintain proper form. A few exercises like sprints and Tabatas will require 90 percent effort and speed, but we'll get to those when we cover the program.

Q. How should I breathe for each movement?

A. For most exercises we'll cover when to breathe in and out, but overall it's a good idea to breathe out when you're exerting the most force (pushing, pulling, etc.) and breathe in on the recovery. Breathing properly is a big part of being able to perform some of the rapid movements we'll be covering in this book, so make sure to focus on breathing rhythmically and not holding your breath during sets.

Q. I was able to follow the program very well early on but am now having trouble doing the required reps. What's going on?

A. Initially, your body goes through a number of changes when you start a new program. Your body will soon begin to adapt to the workouts; you'll notice a plateau once you become used to doing any exercise. This program has been carefully designed to avoid this plateau effect by changing the duration, intensity and workout routine over 90 days. Follow the program as best you can. In the unlikely event you do hit a plateau, continue to follow the plan and eventually there'll be enough change to get you over the hump. Remember, don't overdo it and be sure to take the necessary rest between workouts.

Q. Should I be sore after every workout?

A. Soreness is normal if you're a beginner, have recently changed up your routine or are trying a new activity. The initial soreness should lessen over time; it's not normal to be sore after every workout. If you continue to be sore, you may need to take more days off between workouts.

Q. Will full-body strength training make women bulk up?

A. The bodyweight exercises in this book were selected for men and women to develop lean, shredded bodies. Typically, women don't have the kind of hormones necessary to build huge, bulky muscles. Full-body strength training benefits both men and women by creating leaner tissue and losing any excess fat (by increasing metabolic efficiency), slowing muscle loss (especially in older adults) and decreasing risk for injury.

Q. Will this workout be an effective way to lose weight?

A. The combination of bodyweight strength training with the cardiovascular training from performing supersets (many exercises with no rest in between), Tabatas (20 seconds of intense exercise followed by 10 seconds of rest) and the sprinting involved in the fitness games is the most efficient way for you to lose weight. When paired with balanced nutrition, you'll be firing up your metabolism in as little as 20 minutes a day to burn excess fat and shred your physique.

Q. What is the best time of day to do these workouts?

A. Choosing a time is completely up to your preference. I personally like the feeling of a great morning routine energizing me for the whole day, but I originally conceived this program while working out at lunchtime at the park near my office. After a quick shower at the gym, I was more energized at work in the afternoon after workouts than I was in the morning. The workouts in this book are designed to be done almost anywhere, so pick a time that works for you. You could do sets of exercises while you get ready in the morning or after you get the kids to bed.

Q. Can I combine other workouts with this program?

A. If you're an athlete who needs to train sports-specific skills, then the workouts in this book should be used to supplement that training. If you're hoping to get stronger or more ripped faster by doing extra workouts on "rest days," then you're in danger of overtraining and not letting your muscles rest, recover and grow. For best results, follow the program—rest included—for 90 days.

Q. What's the single best tip you can give to someone about to start this program?

A. Commit the time and effort to do the program right. Often it really helps to have a partner or two (that's how we created the programs!) who'll keep you on track to complete the workouts. Mark workout days on your calendar, or set an alert on your computer or smartphone for the short amount of time the program takes. You can do what Jason and I did— block your calendar from noon to 1 p.m. each day to make sure you get uninterrupted exercise time.

BALANCED NUTRITION

Balanced nutrition is actually pretty simple, but we're bombarded by millions of dollars' worth of advertising touting unhealthy foods. For the most part, we spend very little time really thinking about what we put into our mouths on a daily basis. Sure, we're all busy every day, but a little planning and picking up some healthy snacks can prevent your stomach from steering you into a really unhealthy food choice.

Developing balanced nutrition just requires a little knowledge of your food's nutritional value and some easy planning. Your body constantly adjusts to stay in balance. It may sound like a ridiculous oversimplification but, by eating healthy, balanced foods, you make it that much easier for your body to function at peak condition. Here are my top-10 super-quick tips for assessing your daily food intake.

TIP 1   Keep a food journal for a week. Write down absolutely everything that you put in your belly— water included—for seven days (or longer, if necessary) so you can figure out your patterns. Include time, quantity and how hungry you felt on a scale of 1–10. Make a note about what physical activity you did that day as well; there's usually a correlation between exertion and hunger. The more information you put in your journal, the more data you have to analyze and figure out your patterns.

TIP 2   Don't let yourself get famished. If your stomach is grumbling, there's a good chance you'll overeat or snack on something unhealthy. You're more prone to ignore the unhealthiness of your snack or overdo the portions in your impulse to fill your belly. Eating smaller meals more often throughout the day is the easiest way to combat the tummy grumbles and avoid sabotaging your daily food intake.

TIP 3   Spend more time in the produce aisle of your grocery store. Fresh veggies require a little more effort than grabbing french fries at a drive-through, but one builds healthy bodies and the other builds love handles. Experiment with adding a green pepper to your morning omelet in place of bacon or have an apple instead of a candy bar.

TIP 4   Take a picture of your food and drink before you eat it. This helps you remember what you ate, when you ate it and the portion size. Often, when you're really hungry, you overlook all the extra calories in that meal—the cheese, condiments, bacon, etc. If your food came in a package that has a label, take a picture of that, too. Balanced nutrition starts with knowing the nutritional value of your food. Use those labels to help with planning your protein, carbohydrate, fat and calorie intake.

Shop at the edges of the grocery store. Grocery stores generally keep products that spoil (i.e., have no artificial preservatives) at the exterior edges of the store, leaving the interior for canned goods, processed foods and boxed items. Watch where you're spending the majority of your time and where you're getting the bulk of your calories. General rule: If you get most of your calories from the interior of a grocery store, you need to change your diet.

TIP 5   Drink more water. Soda pop, lemonade, energy drinks, beer—they taste so good and are a huge part of our daily lives. Unfortunately, they're also a huge part of our daily caloric intake. A quick web search shows that the average American consumes approximately 400 calories a day from sugary beverages. Those 146,000 extra calories can translate into as much as 40 pounds of weight gain a year. Here's the great news: If you cut sugary drinks out of your daily fluid intake and drink 2–3 quarts of ice-cold water a day, you'll benefit from cutting hundreds of calories (and chemicals) from your daily intake. Ice-cold water makes your body work harder to warm it to body temperature. In addition, the more hydrated you are, the more often you'll urinate. Each trip to the restroom will force you to get up from your desk and be active. Drinking water also regulates your blood pressure, transports nutrients and keeps all your bodily systems running smoothly.

TIP 6   Eat real foods. The more you can avoid processed foods, the healthier you'll be. Meat, fish, poultry, vegetables, fruits, nuts and seeds don't have nutrition facts labels on them because you know what nutritional value they contain. While I'm not advocating a full-on diet change, the Paleo diets are very effective in helping some individuals get healthier and leaner. I suggest meeting in the middle—fewer processed foods than you eat now and more healthier real foods. If you're vegetarian or gluten intolerant, you'll need to adjust any food intake to meet your dietary restrictions.

"Protein" rhymes with "lean." While the USDA RDA for protein is .36 grams per pound of bodyweight to maintain a healthy diet, to get ripped you need to consume approximately 1 gram of lean protein per pound of your desired weight. In order to do this, you'll need to plan your meals and snacks around protein content first, and these lean proteins will make up about 50% of your daily food intake.

TIP 7   Avoid the extra calories when eating out. When you're eating at home, you know exactly what ingredients are going into your meal. When eating out, you have a lot less knowledge of and control over all the extra calories that get put into that meal. The added butter, salt, sugar and dressing can really add up to make that healthy meal you ordered a calorie and fat bomb. Ask for any dressing on the side and your meats or vegetable cooked "plain" without sauces or butter. Spend a few minutes scanning the menu for healthy choices and make sure to ask your server to help keep them healthy.

It's really that simple. If you can't find a healthy choice, then choose a salad with plenty of veggies (and even some grilled chicken) and make sure you get the dressing on the side. Sometimes it's better to have a salad, leave a little hungry and have a healthy snack at home.

TIP 8   What happens in the pantry doesn't stay in the pantry. The first step is to banish all the unhealthy snack food from your house—if it's not there, you can't snack on it. Sure, you may have fantastic willpower, but when you have a craving and see that bag of chips, you're putting yourself in a predicament for no good reason. Having some fruit in a bowl on the counter works wonders—you see it constantly, you can grab it on the way out the door and you'll also feel guilty if you bought it and allowed it to go bad right under your nose. Celery and carrots last even longer in the fridge than fruit and are always a great snack. A handful of nuts and dried cranberries will go a long way in fueling your body and fending off any cravings for sugary snacks.

TIP 9   Plan your snacks just like your meals. A "snack" absolutely does not have to be something decadent that you need to feel bad about after eating. Actually, snacks play a major role in fueling your body throughout the day. Did you know that your body burns more calories while it's processing food than when you have an empty stomach? Snacks fill in the gap between meals and keep your body burning calories all day long. Plan your snacks by bringing a couple of pieces of fruit to work or on your daily activities. Granola, nuts and dried fruit all travel well. There are plenty of healthy options in energy and nutrition bars, but be aware of the calorie density and nutritional value. If you're (occasionally) eating a meal replacement bar, make sure it's replacing a meal and not a snack. If you have healthy snacks available, you'll make your choices far more easily.

TIP 10   It's all about balance. In order to stay active, build a lean physique, and keep your energy level high, you need to get enough macro and micronutrients and water each day. Macronutrients include fats, proteins and carbohydrates; micronutrients include vitamins and minerals. Your body requires vitamins to regulate its complex chemistry, including that of the digestive and nervous systems. Minerals are the building blocks for bone strength and cardiovascular health. Meats, fruits and vegetables contain plenty of the vitamins and minerals your body needs on a daily basis. Vitamin supplements are also a good way to make sure your body is getting the vital micronutrients it needs.

BEFORE YOU BEGIN

In order to focus on completing this program successfully, it's important to be ready for the challenge and know your limits. When you begin any new exercise program, it's imperative that you talk with your doctor first and make sure you're healthy enough to participate in physical strength training and conditioning.

Once you begin *The Gym-Free Journal* program, perform it at your own pace and within your personal level of fitness. If you feel extremely fatigued or have an uncomfortable level of pain and soreness, take two to three days off from the workout. If the discomfort or pain persists, you should see a health care professional. Due to the nature of a full-body workout routine, you'll be lifting, pushing and pressing your entire bodyweight. Make sure you recognize any physical limitations such as weak or injury-prone joints. It's far more important to be careful with nagging injuries than it is to worry about completing all the exercises in a specified amount of time. Ninety days is an optimum amount of time to get ripped, but not if you ignore the warning signs and hurt yourself.

Some moves will require you to lift your bodyweight on bars, benches, chairs or other objects. Please make sure that the apparatus you're using is sturdy enough to handle more than double your weight. Be smart and safe—don't take any chances with unsafe equipment, and make sure you're properly trained to use any equipment before you start a workout. Always be aware of your surroundings and make sure you have plenty of room to execute moves safely without hitting or tripping over other objects.

WARMING UP & STRETCHING

Properly warming up the body prior to any activity is very important, as is stretching post-workout. Please note that warming up and stretching are two completely different things: A warm-up routine should be done before stretching so that your muscles are more pliable and able to be stretched efficiently. You should not "warm up" by stretching; you simply don't want to push, pull or stretch cold muscles. Prior to warming up, your muscles are significantly less flexible. Think of pulling a rubber band out of a freezer: If you stretch it forcefully before it has a chance to warm up, you'll likely tear it. Stretching cold muscles can cause a significantly higher rate of muscle strains and even injuries to joints that rely on those muscles for alignment.

It's crucial to raise your body temperature prior to beginning a workout. In order to prevent injury, such as a muscle strain, you want to loosen up your muscles and joints before you begin the actual exercise movement. A good warm-up before your workout should slowly raise your core body temperature, heart rate and breathing. Before jumping into the workout, you must increase blood flow to all working areas of the body. This augmented blood flow will transport more oxygen and nutrients to the muscles being worked. The warm-up will also increase the range of motion of your joints.

Another goal is to focus your mental awareness and body proprioception. You've heard that meditation requires being present in the "now." The same is true for a demanding exercise routine. Being totally present and focused will help you perform better and avoid injury.

A warm-up should consist of light physical activity (such as walking, jogging, stationary biking or jumping jacks) and only take 5–10 minutes to complete. Your individual fitness level and the activity determine how hard and how long you should go but, generally speaking, the average person should build up to a light sweat during warm-ups. You want to prepare your body for activity, not fatigue it. A warm-up should be done in these stages:

Gentle Mobility: Easy movements that get your joints moving freely, like standing arm raises, arm and shoulder circles, neck rotations, and trunk twists.

Pulse Raising: Gentle, progressive, aerobic activity that starts the process of raising your heart rate, like jumping jacks, skipping rope or running in place.

Specific Mobility: This begins working the joints and muscles that will be used during the activity. Perform dynamic movements to prepare your body for your upcoming full-body workout. These movements are done more rapidly than the gentle mobility movements—envision a swimmer before a race or a weightlifter before a big lift. Dynamic movements should raise the heart rate, loosen specific joints and muscles, and get you motivated for your workout.

Stretching should generally be done after a workout. It'll help you reduce soreness from the workout, increase range of motion and flexibility within a joint or muscle, and prepare your body for any future workouts. Stretching immediately post-exercise while your muscles are still warm allows your muscles to return to their full range of motion (which gives you more flexibility gains) and reduces the chance of injury or fatigue in the hours or days after an intense workout. It's important to remember that even when you're warm and loose, you should never "bounce" during stretching. Keep your movements slow and controlled.

To recap, you should warm up for 5–10 minutes, perform your workout, and then stretch for 5–10 minutes. We've included a few warm-up exercises and stretches that specifically target the muscles used in each workout (see page 231).

AVOIDING INJURIES

As I covered earlier in the FAQs (page 14), bodyweight strength training combined with cardiovascular exercises is the most efficient way to build strength and develop a lean, ripped physique. Let's be honest, though; none of us are perfect. Due to years of improper posture, sports injuries or even weak musculature, we all have imbalances that can affect proper form and even put us on the fast track to injury. In addition, jumping into a new exercise routine too quickly or doing the exercises with improper form can exacerbate any pre-existing injury.

It's very important that you focus on proper form and utilize the proper muscles to complete each exercise. This means no cheating by arching your back on push-ups or swinging your legs on pull-ups. You're only cheating yourself; every proper-form rep just gets you closer to ripped! If you have a pre-existing condition like rotator cuff soreness or a muscular imbalance, take your time and work your way up slowly while focusing on training with good form. If pain or soreness persists, please see a medical professional.

Speaking of professionals, remember that no one expects you to be a pro at every movement. Some exercises may come naturally while others feel completely foreign. I personally fight with keeping my shoulders level when performing pull-ups. All you can do is keep working on perfecting the form and get stronger along the way. Don't give up and sit out an exercise if you can't do it—make the investment in yourself and learn the proper form for each move. You'll only reap the benefits.

LISTEN TO YOUR BODY

You should be able to tell how you're doing on a strength and conditioning program like this one by tuning in to your body. Take it easy and be smart about determining what's normal soreness from a workout and what's a nagging injury that you're aggravating. If you think it's the latter, take a few extra days off and see if the soreness passes. If it doesn't, you should see a medical professional. Throughout the routine, you should expect to experience mild soreness and fatigue, especially when you're just getting started. The feeling of your muscles being "pumped" and the fatigue of an exhausting workout should be expected. These are positive feelings.

On the other hand, any sharp pain, muscle spasm or numbness is a warning sign that you need to stop and not push yourself any harder. Some small muscle groups may fatigue more quickly because they're often overlooked in other workouts. Your hands and forearms are doing a tremendous amount of work and can easily tire out. If you feel you can't grip or support yourself with your hands anymore, take a rest. It's far better than slipping and getting hurt.

Here are a few other symptoms to watch for: sore elbows, shoulder (rotator cuff) pain and stiff neck. Sore elbows are usually a sign that you're locking out your elbows when your arms are fully extended; remember to keep a slight bend in your elbows. Pain in the rotator cuff can be caused by poor form or a hand position that is too wide while doing pull-ups or push-ups. A stiff neck can result from straining your neck throughout the movement; try to keep your neck loose and flexible. If any of these pains persists, it's imperative that you seek medical advice.

A WORD ABOUT INTENSITY

The higher the level of intensity you put into the workout, the more you'll reap the benefits. Moving from exercise to exercise quickly during supersets, finishing every rep with proper form, putting the hammer down on sprints and speedwork and executing each workout from start to finish is the most efficient way to develop the ripped body you want. *The Gym-Free Journal* workouts are progressive, which means they'll build and get harder over time. All of the workouts—including the initial ones—are challenging, and it's up to you to complete the program at your own intensity. If you sleepwalk through the movements and slog from one exercise to the next, you're only cheating yourself. *The Gym-Free Journal* is a commitment of about 20 minutes of intense workout 3 days a week. Throw in an hour of physical activity over the weekend and your weekly commitment is only about 2 hours—that's less than some people wait in line per week at their local coffee shop. Stay focused and keep the intensity high throughout your workouts. Don't forget to hydrate and breathe properly, too!

PART 2:
THE PROGRAM

THE WORKOUT JOURNAL

Welcome to *The Gym-Free Journal* workouts! Since this book and program are designed to fit the majority of beginner and intermediate athletes of any age, sex, size, and previous athletic ability, there's no "one size fits all" program that will work right out of the box. So, this is where your effort and intensity comes in!

Consider this program "some assembly required" if it doesn't fit your ability and goals right off the bat. If it's too hard, then complete one set per day for the first week or two and build your way up to completing the entire Week 1 before you move on to Week 2. Be sure to use any assistance as needed—use an exercise band or chair for pull-ups and chin-ups, steady yourself by holding onto a bar or wall for squats and lunges, perform push-ups on your knees or use the wall variation. Use the tools at your disposal to give you an edge and make each workout successful so you can keep coming back and progressively get stronger and fitter to complete every workout.

Is the program too easy? Well, there's a simple fix for that: intensity! Move from each exercise to the next with little or no break and even cut the rest periods down to zero if you feel like the required reps are too low. The faster you do it—with good form, of course—the harder it'll be. Ignore the word "assisted" with the pull-ups and, if needed, add an additional set or two (or even three) to make each workout a gasser. As you progress through the weeks, this will eventually become much more difficult, if not impossible, to keep up.

For the cardio sections, you can use an elliptical, treadmill, or stationary bike, get in the pool for a swim, hit the sidewalk or trails for a run, or any number of other athletic pursuits that require a mix of low- and high-intensity movements and get your heart pumping for the required time in the program. Be creative and break out a jump rope, chase after your dog, run up some stairs and walk back down. Pick something that works for your schedule and surroundings.

USING THE CHARTS

Monday, Wednesday and Friday are your workout days. On these pages, write down how many reps of a certain movement you actually completed, how much weight you lifted, or how long you held an exercise for. At the bottom of each workout chart, there's space for you to make notes if you want. It can be helpful to write down how you're feeling before, during or after a workout. Did you wake up feeling sluggish but the workout pumped up your energy? Are you feeling hungry in the middle of a workout? Over time, these can all be indicators of your progress, and you can adjust your habits based on any trends you're seeing. Maybe you need to get more sleep or eat more protein in your daily snacks.

Rest days have been left blank, but be sure to note anything you did those days that might affect future workouts—a hike you went on with friends, or a big meeting that kept you sitting down all day. Maybe note whether you're feeling like you're dying to work out and like resting is the worst. Just be sure to resist the temptation to do a few squats or burpees! These rest days are built in to the program for a reason, and they'll help you be stronger in the long run.

Both workout and non-workout days include a nutrition log. What you eat is critical to achieving your fitness goals, whether you want to lose weight, gain muscle, or just have an easier time chasing after your dog. There's space to note calories and quantities of macronutrients, but the most important thing is just to be honest with yourself about the things you're putting in your body. Just like the workout log, look for trends in how your eating affects your body and mind, and how they work while you exercise. After all, that's the point of the journal: to figure out what you need and what works best for your body.

Rest and rehydrate as needed between sets; maintain as high an intensity as possible between moves while maintaining proper form.

MONDAY (DAY 1)

5–10 min	WARM-UP *page 231*	

SET 1		Reps / Time / Weight
4 reps	PUSH-UPS *page 214*	
6 reps	SQUATS *page 220*	
30 sec	PLANK *page 223*	
3 reps	ASSISTED CHIN-UPS *page 216*	

SET 2		Reps / Time / Weight
5 reps	PUSH-UPS *page 214*	
5 reps	LUNGES EACH LEG *page 221*	
3 reps	ASSISTED PULL-UPS *page 216*	
8 reps	IN & OUTS *page 224*	

SET 3		Reps / Time / Weight
10 reps	WOOD CHOPS *page 225*	
16 reps	MARCHING TWISTS *page 225*	
8 reps	MOUNTAIN CLIMBERS *page 226*	
10 min	CARDIO	
5–10 min	STRETCH *page 231*	

NOTES

MONDAY (DAY 1)

BREAKFAST	Calories:	Protein:	Carbs:	Fat:

SNACK 1	Calories:	Protein:	Carbs:	Fat:

LUNCH	Calories:	Protein:	Carbs:	Fat:

DINNER	Calories:	Protein:	Carbs:	Fat:

SNACK 2	Calories:	Protein:	Carbs:	Fat:

PRE-WORKOUT SNACK	Calories:	Protein:	Carbs:	Fat:

POST-WORKOUT SNACK	Calories:	Protein:	Carbs:	Fat:

TUESDAY (DAY 2)

REST

NOTES

TUESDAY (DAY 2)

BREAKFAST	Calories:	Protein:	Carbs:	Fat:

SNACK 1	Calories:	Protein:	Carbs:	Fat:

LUNCH	Calories:	Protein:	Carbs:	Fat:

DINNER	Calories:	Protein:	Carbs:	Fat:

SNACK 2	Calories:	Protein:	Carbs:	Fat:

PRE-WORKOUT SNACK	Calories:	Protein:	Carbs:	Fat:

POST-WORKOUT SNACK	Calories:	Protein:	Carbs:	Fat:

WEDNESDAY (DAY 3)

5–10 min	WARM-UP *page 231*	

SET I		Reps / Time / Weight
3 reps	PUSH-UPS *page 214*	
20 sec	PLANK *page 223*	
10 reps	MOUNTAIN CLIMBERS *page 226*	
2 reps	ASSISTED PULL-UPS *page 216*	

SET 2		Reps / Time / Weight
6 reps	LUNGES WITH TWIST EACH LEG *page 222*	
10 reps	WOOD CHOPS *page 225*	
18 reps	MARCHING TWISTS *page 225*	
8 reps	SQUATS *page 220*	

SET 3		Reps / Time / Weight
3 reps	ASSISTED CHIN-UPS *page 216*	
8 reps	HANGING LEG RAISES *page 218*	
8 reps	REVERSE CRUNCHES *page 218*	
10 min	CARDIO	
5–10 min	STRETCH *page 231*	

NOTES

WEDNESDAY (DAY 3)

BREAKFAST	Calories:	Protein:	Carbs:	Fat:

SNACK 1	Calories:	Protein:	Carbs:	Fat:

LUNCH	Calories:	Protein:	Carbs:	Fat:

DINNER	Calories:	Protein:	Carbs:	Fat:

SNACK 2	Calories:	Protein:	Carbs:	Fat:

PRE-WORKOUT SNACK	Calories:	Protein:	Carbs:	Fat:

POST-WORKOUT SNACK	Calories:	Protein:	Carbs:	Fat:

THURSDAY (DAY 4)

REST

NOTES

THURSDAY (DAY 4)

BREAKFAST	Calories:	Protein:	Carbs:	Fat:

SNACK I	Calories:	Protein:	Carbs:	Fat:

LUNCH	Calories:	Protein:	Carbs:	Fat:

DINNER	Calories:	Protein:	Carbs:	Fat:

SNACK 2	Calories:	Protein:	Carbs:	Fat:

PRE-WORKOUT SNACK	Calories:	Protein:	Carbs:	Fat:

POST-WORKOUT SNACK	Calories:	Protein:	Carbs:	Fat:

FRIDAY (DAY 5)

5–10 min	WARM-UP *page 231*	

SET 1		Reps / Time / Weight
3 reps	ASSISTED PULL-UPS *page 216*	
5 reps	PUSH-UPS *page 214*	
8 reps	SQUATS WITH MEDICINE BALL *page 221*	
12 reps	MOUNTAIN CLIMBERS *page 226*	

SET 2		Reps / Time / Weight
10 reps	HANGING LEG RAISES *page 218*	
6 reps	LUNGES WITH TWIST EACH LEG *page 222*	
5 reps	PUSH-UPS *page 214*	
10 reps	IN & OUTS *page 224*	

SET 2		Reps / Time / Weight
3 reps	ASSISTED CHIN-UPS *page 216*	
12 reps	WOOD CHOPS *page 225*	
20 reps	MARCHING TWISTS *page 225*	
10 min	CARDIO	
5–10 min	STRETCH *page 231*	

NOTES

FRIDAY (DAY 5)

BREAKFAST	Calories:	Protein:	Carbs:	Fat:

SNACK I	Calories:	Protein:	Carbs:	Fat:

LUNCH	Calories:	Protein:	Carbs:	Fat:

DINNER	Calories:	Protein:	Carbs:	Fat:

SNACK 2	Calories:	Protein:	Carbs:	Fat:

PRE-WORKOUT SNACK	Calories:	Protein:	Carbs:	Fat:

POST-WORKOUT SNACK	Calories:	Protein:	Carbs:	Fat:

SATURDAY (DAY 6)

REST

NOTES

SATURDAY (DAY 6)

BREAKFAST	Calories:	Protein:	Carbs:	Fat:

SNACK 1	Calories:	Protein:	Carbs:	Fat:

LUNCH	Calories:	Protein:	Carbs:	Fat:

DINNER	Calories:	Protein:	Carbs:	Fat:

SNACK 2	Calories:	Protein:	Carbs:	Fat:

PRE-WORKOUT SNACK	Calories:	Protein:	Carbs:	Fat:

POST-WORKOUT SNACK	Calories:	Protein:	Carbs:	Fat:

SUNDAY (DAY 7)

REST

NOTES

SUNDAY (DAY 7)

BREAKFAST	Calories:	Protein:	Carbs:	Fat:

SNACK 1	Calories:	Protein:	Carbs:	Fat:

LUNCH	Calories:	Protein:	Carbs:	Fat:

DINNER	Calories:	Protein:	Carbs:	Fat:

SNACK 2	Calories:	Protein:	Carbs:	Fat:

PRE-WORKOUT SNACK	Calories:	Protein:	Carbs:	Fat:

POST-WORKOUT SNACK	Calories:	Protein:	Carbs:	Fat:

MONDAY (DAY 8)

5–10 min	WARM-UP *page 231*	

SET I		Reps / Time / Weight
5 reps	ASSISTED CHIN-UPS *page 216*	
10 reps	SQUATS *page 220*	
8 reps	PUSH-UPS *page 214*	
30 sec	PLANK *page 223*	

SET 2		Reps / Time / Weight
14 reps	WOOD CHOPS *page 225*	
12 reps	MOUNTAIN CLIMBERS *page 226*	
20 reps	MARCHING TWISTS *page 225*	
12 reps	JUMPING JACKS *page 227*	

SET I		Reps / Time / Weight
6 reps	PUSH-UPS *page 214*	
30 sec	PLANK *page 223*	
15 sec	SIDE PLANK EACH SIDE *page 224*	
10 reps	REVERSE CRUNCHES *page 218*	
10 min	CARDIO	
5–10 min	STRETCH *page 231*	

NOTES

MONDAY (DAY 8)

BREAKFAST	Calories:	Protein:	Carbs:	Fat:

SNACK 1	Calories:	Protein:	Carbs:	Fat:

LUNCH	Calories:	Protein:	Carbs:	Fat:

DINNER	Calories:	Protein:	Carbs:	Fat:

SNACK 2	Calories:	Protein:	Carbs:	Fat:

PRE-WORKOUT SNACK	Calories:	Protein:	Carbs:	Fat:

POST-WORKOUT SNACK	Calories:	Protein:	Carbs:	Fat:

TUESDAY (DAY 9)

REST

NOTES

TUESDAY (DAY 9)

BREAKFAST	Calories:	Protein:	Carbs:	Fat:

SNACK 1	Calories:	Protein:	Carbs:	Fat:

LUNCH	Calories:	Protein:	Carbs:	Fat:

DINNER	Calories:	Protein:	Carbs:	Fat:

SNACK 2	Calories:	Protein:	Carbs:	Fat:

PRE-WORKOUT SNACK	Calories:	Protein:	Carbs:	Fat:

POST-WORKOUT SNACK	Calories:	Protein:	Carbs:	Fat:

WEDNESDAY (DAY 10)

5–10 min	WARM-UP *page 231*	

SET 1		Reps / Time / Weight
6 reps	ASSISTED PULL-UPS *page 216*	
5 reps	PUSH-UPS *page 214*	
8 reps	SQUATS WITH MEDICINE BALL *page 221*	
10 reps	MOUNTAIN CLIMBERS *page 226*	

SET 2		Reps / Time / Weight
10 reps	HANGING LEG RAISES *page 218*	
6 reps	LUNGES WITH TWIST EACH LEG *page 222*	
5 reps	PUSH-UPS *page 214*	
10 reps	IN & OUTS *page 224*	

SET 3		Reps / Time / Weight
8 reps	PUSH-UPS *page 214*	
11 reps	SQUATS *page 220*	
30 sec	PLANK *page 223*	
6 reps	ASSISTED CHIN-UPS *page 216*	
10 min	CARDIO	
5–10 min	STRETCH *page 231*	

NOTES

WEDNESDAY (DAY 10)

BREAKFAST	Calories:	Protein:	Carbs:	Fat:

SNACK 1	Calories:	Protein:	Carbs:	Fat:

LUNCH	Calories:	Protein:	Carbs:	Fat:

DINNER	Calories:	Protein:	Carbs:	Fat:

SNACK 2	Calories:	Protein:	Carbs:	Fat:

PRE-WORKOUT SNACK	Calories:	Protein:	Carbs:	Fat:

POST-WORKOUT SNACK	Calories:	Protein:	Carbs:	Fat:

THURSDAY (DAY 11)

REST

NOTES

THURSDAY (DAY 11)

BREAKFAST	Calories:	Protein:	Carbs:	Fat:

SNACK 1	Calories:	Protein:	Carbs:	Fat:

LUNCH	Calories:	Protein:	Carbs:	Fat:

DINNER	Calories:	Protein:	Carbs:	Fat:

SNACK 2	Calories:	Protein:	Carbs:	Fat:

PRE-WORKOUT SNACK	Calories:	Protein:	Carbs:	Fat:

POST-WORKOUT SNACK	Calories:	Protein:	Carbs:	Fat:

FRIDAY (DAY 12)		
5–10 min	WARM-UP *page 231*	
SET 1		Reps / Time / Weight
8 reps	PUSH-UPS *page 214*	
11 reps	SQUATS *page 220*	
30 sec	PLANK *page 223*	
6 reps	ASSISTED CHIN-UPS *page 216*	
SET 2		Reps / Time / Weight
8 reps	PUSH-UPS *page 214*	
8 reps	LUNGES WITH TWIST EACH LEG *page 222*	
2 reps	PULL-UPS *page 216*	
10 reps	IN & OUTS *page 224*	
SET 3		Reps / Time / Weight
14 reps	WOOD CHOPS *page 225*	
20 reps	MARCHING TWISTS *page 225*	
12 reps	MOUNTAIN CLIMBERS *page 226*	
12 reps	JUMPING JACKS *page 227*	
10 min	CARDIO	
5–10 min	STRETCH *page 231*	

NOTES

FRIDAY (DAY 12)

BREAKFAST	Calories:	Protein:	Carbs:	Fat:

SNACK 1	Calories:	Protein:	Carbs:	Fat:

LUNCH	Calories:	Protein:	Carbs:	Fat:

DINNER	Calories:	Protein:	Carbs:	Fat:

SNACK 2	Calories:	Protein:	Carbs:	Fat:

PRE-WORKOUT SNACK	Calories:	Protein:	Carbs:	Fat:

POST-WORKOUT SNACK	Calories:	Protein:	Carbs:	Fat:

SATURDAY (DAY 13)

REST

NOTES

SATURDAY (DAY 13)

BREAKFAST	Calories:	Protein:	Carbs:	Fat:

SNACK 1	Calories:	Protein:	Carbs:	Fat:

LUNCH	Calories:	Protein:	Carbs:	Fat:

DINNER	Calories:	Protein:	Carbs:	Fat:

SNACK 2	Calories:	Protein:	Carbs:	Fat:

PRE-WORKOUT SNACK	Calories:	Protein:	Carbs:	Fat:

POST-WORKOUT SNACK	Calories:	Protein:	Carbs:	Fat:

SUNDAY (DAY 14)

REST

SUNDAY (DAY 14)

BREAKFAST	Calories:	Protein:	Carbs:	Fat:

SNACK 1	Calories:	Protein:	Carbs:	Fat:

LUNCH	Calories:	Protein:	Carbs:	Fat:

DINNER	Calories:	Protein:	Carbs:	Fat:

SNACK 2	Calories:	Protein:	Carbs:	Fat:

PRE-WORKOUT SNACK	Calories:	Protein:	Carbs:	Fat:

POST-WORKOUT SNACK	Calories:	Protein:	Carbs:	Fat:

MONDAY (DAY 15)

5–10 min	WARM-UP *page 231*	
SET I		Reps / Time / Weight
6 reps	ASSISTED PULL-UPS *page 216*	
8 reps	PUSH-UPS *page 214*	
12 reps	SQUATS WITH MEDICINE BALL *page 221*	
14 reps	MOUNTAIN CLIMBERS *page 226*	
SET 2		Reps / Time / Weight
12 reps	HANGING LEG RAISES *page 218*	
8 reps	LUNGES WITH TWIST EACH LEG *page 222*	
8 reps	PUSH-UPS *page 214*	
10 reps	REVERSE CRUNCHES *page 218*	
SET 2		Reps / Time / Weight
3 reps	CHIN-UPS *page 216*	
14 reps	WOOD CHOPS *page 225*	
20 reps	MARCHING TWISTS *page 225*	
45 sec	PLANK *page 223*	
10 min	CARDIO	
5–10 min	STRETCH *page 231*	

NOTES

MONDAY (DAY 15)

BREAKFAST	Calories:	Protein:	Carbs:	Fat:

SNACK 1	Calories:	Protein:	Carbs:	Fat:

LUNCH	Calories:	Protein:	Carbs:	Fat:

DINNER	Calories:	Protein:	Carbs:	Fat:

SNACK 2	Calories:	Protein:	Carbs:	Fat:

PRE-WORKOUT SNACK	Calories:	Protein:	Carbs:	Fat:

POST-WORKOUT SNACK	Calories:	Protein:	Carbs:	Fat:

TUESDAY (DAY 16)

REST

NOTES

TUESDAY (DAY 16)

BREAKFAST	Calories:	Protein:	Carbs:	Fat:

SNACK 1	Calories:	Protein:	Carbs:	Fat:

LUNCH	Calories:	Protein:	Carbs:	Fat:

DINNER	Calories:	Protein:	Carbs:	Fat:

SNACK 2	Calories:	Protein:	Carbs:	Fat:

PRE-WORKOUT SNACK	Calories:	Protein:	Carbs:	Fat:

POST-WORKOUT SNACK	Calories:	Protein:	Carbs:	Fat:

WEDNESDAY (DAY 17)

5–10 min	WARM-UP *page 231*	

SET 1		Reps / Time / Weight
12 reps	HANGING LEG RAISES *page 218*	
8 reps	LUNGES WITH TWIST EACH LEG *page 222*	
9 reps	PUSH-UPS *page 214*	
12 reps	IN & OUTS *page 224*	

SET 2		Reps / Time / Weight
3 reps	PULL-UPS *page 216*	
8 reps	PUSH-UPS *page 214*	
14 reps	SQUATS WITH MEDICINE BALL *page 221*	
16 reps	MOUNTAIN CLIMBERS *page 226*	

SET 3		Reps / Time / Weight
3 reps	CHIN-UPS *page 216*	
16 reps	WOOD CHOPS *page 225*	
20 reps	MARCHING TWISTS *page 225*	
12 reps	SQUATS *page 220*	
10 min	CARDIO	
5–10 min	STRETCH *page 231*	

NOTES

WEDNESDAY (DAY 17)

BREAKFAST	Calories:	Protein:	Carbs:	Fat:

SNACK I	Calories:	Protein:	Carbs:	Fat:

LUNCH	Calories:	Protein:	Carbs:	Fat:

DINNER	Calories:	Protein:	Carbs:	Fat:

SNACK 2	Calories:	Protein:	Carbs:	Fat:

PRE-WORKOUT SNACK	Calories:	Protein:	Carbs:	Fat:

POST-WORKOUT SNACK	Calories:	Protein:	Carbs:	Fat:

THURSDAY (DAY 18)

REST

NOTES

THURSDAY (DAY 18)

BREAKFAST	Calories:	Protein:	Carbs:	Fat:

SNACK 1	Calories:	Protein:	Carbs:	Fat:

LUNCH	Calories:	Protein:	Carbs:	Fat:

DINNER	Calories:	Protein:	Carbs:	Fat:

SNACK 2	Calories:	Protein:	Carbs:	Fat:

PRE-WORKOUT SNACK	Calories:	Protein:	Carbs:	Fat:

POST-WORKOUT SNACK	Calories:	Protein:	Carbs:	Fat:

FRIDAY (DAY 19)

5–10 min	WARM-UP *page 231*	

SET I		Reps / Time / Weight
4 reps	CHIN-UPS *page 216*	
14 reps	HANGING LEG RAISES *page 218*	
9 reps	LUNGES WITH TWIST EACH LEG *page 222*	
8 reps	PUSH-UPS *page 214*	

SET 2		Reps / Time / Weight
3 reps	PULL-UPS *page 216*	
16 reps	SQUATS *page 220*	
45 sec	PLANK *page 223*	
8 reps	PUSH-UPS *page 214*	

SET 3		Reps / Time / Weight
3 reps	CHIN-UPS *page 216*	
14 reps	REVERSE CRUNCHES *page 218*	
16 reps	MOUNTAIN CLIMBERS *page 226*	
18 reps	WOOD CHOPS *page 225*	
10 min	CARDIO	
5–10 min	STRETCH *page 231*	

NOTES

FRIDAY (DAY 19)

BREAKFAST	Calories:	Protein:	Carbs:	Fat:

SNACK 1	Calories:	Protein:	Carbs:	Fat:

LUNCH	Calories:	Protein:	Carbs:	Fat:

DINNER	Calories:	Protein:	Carbs:	Fat:

SNACK 2	Calories:	Protein:	Carbs:	Fat:

PRE-WORKOUT SNACK	Calories:	Protein:	Carbs:	Fat:

POST-WORKOUT SNACK	Calories:	Protein:	Carbs:	Fat:

SATURDAY (DAY 20)

REST

NOTES

SATURDAY (DAY 20)

BREAKFAST	Calories:	Protein:	Carbs:	Fat:

SNACK 1	Calories:	Protein:	Carbs:	Fat:

LUNCH	Calories:	Protein:	Carbs:	Fat:

DINNER	Calories:	Protein:	Carbs:	Fat:

SNACK 2	Calories:	Protein:	Carbs:	Fat:

PRE-WORKOUT SNACK	Calories:	Protein:	Carbs:	Fat:

POST-WORKOUT SNACK	Calories:	Protein:	Carbs:	Fat:

SUNDAY (DAY 21)

REST

NOTES

SUNDAY (DAY 21)

BREAKFAST	Calories:	Protein:	Carbs:	Fat:

SNACK 1	Calories:	Protein:	Carbs:	Fat:

LUNCH	Calories:	Protein:	Carbs:	Fat:

DINNER	Calories:	Protein:	Carbs:	Fat:

SNACK 2	Calories:	Protein:	Carbs:	Fat:

PRE-WORKOUT SNACK	Calories:	Protein:	Carbs:	Fat:

POST-WORKOUT SNACK	Calories:	Protein:	Carbs:	Fat:

MONDAY (DAY 22)

5–10 min	WARM-UP *page 231*	

SET I		Reps / Time / Weight
5 reps	CHIN-UPS *page 216*	
10 reps	SQUATS *page 220*	
10 reps	PUSH-UPS *page 214*	
30 sec	PLANK *page 223*	

SET 2		Reps / Time / Weight
4 reps	PULL-UPS *page 216*	
10 reps	LUNGES EACH LEG *page 221*	
9 reps	NARROW PUSH-UPS *page 214*	
5 reps	V-SITS *page 217*	

SET 3		Reps / Time / Weight
5 reps	CHIN-UPS *page 216*	
10 reps	SQUATS *page 220*	
7 reps	PUSH-UPS *page 214*	
10 reps	IN & OUTS *page 224*	
12 min	CARDIO	
5–10 min	STRETCH *page 231*	

NOTES

MONDAY (DAY 22)

BREAKFAST	Calories:	Protein:	Carbs:	Fat:

SNACK 1	Calories:	Protein:	Carbs:	Fat:

LUNCH	Calories:	Protein:	Carbs:	Fat:

DINNER	Calories:	Protein:	Carbs:	Fat:

SNACK 2	Calories:	Protein:	Carbs:	Fat:

PRE-WORKOUT SNACK	Calories:	Protein:	Carbs:	Fat:

POST-WORKOUT SNACK	Calories:	Protein:	Carbs:	Fat:

TUESDAY (DAY 23)

REST

NOTES

TUESDAY (DAY 23)

BREAKFAST	Calories:	Protein:	Carbs:	Fat:

SNACK 1	Calories:	Protein:	Carbs:	Fat:

LUNCH	Calories:	Protein:	Carbs:	Fat:

DINNER	Calories:	Protein:	Carbs:	Fat:

SNACK 2	Calories:	Protein:	Carbs:	Fat:

PRE-WORKOUT SNACK	Calories:	Protein:	Carbs:	Fat:

POST-WORKOUT SNACK	Calories:	Protein:	Carbs:	Fat:

WEDNESDAY (DAY 24)

5–10 min	WARM-UP *page 231*	
SET I		REPS/TIME/WEIGHT
6 reps	PULL-UPS *page 216*	
12 reps	SQUATS *page 220*	
10 reps	PUSH-UPS *page 214*	
35 sec	PLANK *page 223*	
SET 2		
5 reps	CHIN-UPS *page 216*	
10 reps	LUNGES EACH LEG *page 221*	
7 reps	DIAMOND PUSH-UPS *page 214*	
16 reps	SUPERMANS *page 219*	
SET 3		
5 reps	PULL-UPS *page 216*	
12 reps	SQUATS *page 220*	
10 reps	PUSH-UPS *page 214*	
20 reps	MASON TWISTS *page 226*	
12 min	CARDIO	
5–10 min	STRETCH *page 231*	

NOTES

WEDNESDAY (DAY 24)

BREAKFAST	Calories:	Protein:	Carbs:	Fat:

SNACK 1	Calories:	Protein:	Carbs:	Fat:

LUNCH	Calories:	Protein:	Carbs:	Fat:

DINNER	Calories:	Protein:	Carbs:	Fat:

SNACK 2	Calories:	Protein:	Carbs:	Fat:

PRE-WORKOUT SNACK	Calories:	Protein:	Carbs:	Fat:

POST-WORKOUT SNACK	Calories:	Protein:	Carbs:	Fat:

THURSDAY (DAY 25)

REST

NOTES

THURSDAY (DAY 25)

BREAKFAST	Calories:	Protein:	Carbs:	Fat:

SNACK 1	Calories:	Protein:	Carbs:	Fat:

LUNCH	Calories:	Protein:	Carbs:	Fat:

DINNER	Calories:	Protein:	Carbs:	Fat:

SNACK 2	Calories:	Protein:	Carbs:	Fat:

PRE-WORKOUT SNACK	Calories:	Protein:	Carbs:	Fat:

POST-WORKOUT SNACK	Calories:	Protein:	Carbs:	Fat:

FRIDAY (DAY 26)

5–10 min	WARM-UP *page 231*	

SET 1		Reps / Time / Weight
6 reps	CHIN-UPS *page 216*	
12 reps	SQUATS *page 220*	
12 reps	PUSH-UPS *page 214*	
40 sec	PLANK *page 223*	

SET 2		Reps / Time / Weight
6 reps	PULL-UPS *page 216*	
11 res	LUNGES EACH LEG *page 221*	
10 reps	DIAMOND PUSH-UPS *page 214*	
7 reps	HANGING LEG RAISES *page 218*	

SET 3		Reps / Time / Weight
6 reps	CHIN-UPS *page 216*	
12 reps	SQUATS *page 220*	
12 reps	PUSH-UPS *page 214*	
10 reps	IN & OUTS *page 224*	
12 min	CARDIO	
5–10 min	STRETCH *page 231*	

NOTES

FRIDAY (DAY 26)

BREAKFAST	Calories:	Protein:	Carbs:	Fat:

SNACK 1	Calories:	Protein:	Carbs:	Fat:

LUNCH	Calories:	Protein:	Carbs:	Fat:

DINNER	Calories:	Protein:	Carbs:	Fat:

SNACK 2	Calories:	Protein:	Carbs:	Fat:

PRE-WORKOUT SNACK	Calories:	Protein:	Carbs:	Fat:

POST-WORKOUT SNACK	Calories:	Protein:	Carbs:	Fat:

SATURDAY (DAY 27)

REST

NOTES

SATURDAY (DAY 27)

BREAKFAST	Calories:	Protein:	Carbs:	Fat:

SNACK 1	Calories:	Protein:	Carbs:	Fat:

LUNCH	Calories:	Protein:	Carbs:	Fat:

DINNER	Calories:	Protein:	Carbs:	Fat:

SNACK 2	Calories:	Protein:	Carbs:	Fat:

PRE-WORKOUT SNACK	Calories:	Protein:	Carbs:	Fat:

POST-WORKOUT SNACK	Calories:	Protein:	Carbs:	Fat:

SUNDAY (DAY 28)

REST

NOTES

SUNDAY (DAY 28)

BREAKFAST	Calories:	Protein:	Carbs:	Fat:

SNACK I	Calories:	Protein:	Carbs:	Fat:

LUNCH	Calories:	Protein:	Carbs:	Fat:

DINNER	Calories:	Protein:	Carbs:	Fat:

SNACK 2	Calories:	Protein:	Carbs:	Fat:

PRE-WORKOUT SNACK	Calories:	Protein:	Carbs:	Fat:

POST-WORKOUT SNACK	Calories:	Protein:	Carbs:	Fat:

MONDAY (DAY 29)

5–10 min	WARM-UP *page 231*	
SET 1		Reps / Time / Weight
7 reps	PULL-UPS *page 216*	
12 reps	SQUATS *page 220*	
12 reps	PUSH-UPS *page 214*	
45 sec	PLANK *page 223*	
SET 2		Reps / Time / Weight
7 reps	CHIN-UPS *page 216*	
12 reps	LUNGES EACH LEG *page 221*	
10 reps	NARROW PUSH-UPS *page 214*	
7 reps	SUPERMANS *page 219*	
SET 3		Reps / Time / Weight
7 reps	CHIN-UPS *page 216*	
12 reps	SQUATS *page 220*	
10 reps	PUSH-UPS *page 214*	
8 reps	HANGING LEG RAISES *page 218*	
14 min	CARDIO	
5–10 min	STRETCH *page 231*	

NOTES

MONDAY (DAY 29)

BREAKFAST	Calories:	Protein:	Carbs:	Fat:

SNACK 1	Calories:	Protein:	Carbs:	Fat:

LUNCH	Calories:	Protein:	Carbs:	Fat:

DINNER	Calories:	Protein:	Carbs:	Fat:

SNACK 2	Calories:	Protein:	Carbs:	Fat:

PRE-WORKOUT SNACK	Calories:	Protein:	Carbs:	Fat:

POST-WORKOUT SNACK	Calories:	Protein:	Carbs:	Fat:

TUESDAY (DAY 30)

REST

NOTES

TUESDAY (DAY 30)

BREAKFAST	Calories:	Protein:	Carbs:	Fat:

SNACK I	Calories:	Protein:	Carbs:	Fat:

LUNCH	Calories:	Protein:	Carbs:	Fat:

DINNER	Calories:	Protein:	Carbs:	Fat:

SNACK 2	Calories:	Protein:	Carbs:	Fat:

PRE-WORKOUT SNACK	Calories:	Protein:	Carbs:	Fat:

POST-WORKOUT SNACK	Calories:	Protein:	Carbs:	Fat:

WEDNESDAY (DAY 31)

5–10 min	WARM-UP *page 231*	

SET 1		Reps / Time / Weight
7 reps	CHIN-UPS *page 216*	
12 reps	SQUATS *page 220*	
13 reps	PUSH-UPS *page 214*	
10 reps	HANGING LEG RAISES *page 218*	

SET 2		Reps / Time / Weight
7 reps	PULL-UPS *page 216*	
10 reps	WOOD CHOPS *page 225*	
10 reps	PUSH-UPS *page 214*	
20 reps	MASON TWISTS *page 226*	

SET 3		Reps / Time / Weight
6 reps	PULL-UPS *page 216*	
12 reps	LUNGES PER LEG *page 221*	
12 reps	PUSH-UPS *page 214*	
7 reps	V-SITS *page 217*	
14 min	CARDIO	
5–10 min	STRETCH *page 231*	

NOTES

WEDNESDAY (DAY 31)

BREAKFAST	Calories:	Protein:	Carbs:	Fat:

SNACK I	Calories:	Protein:	Carbs:	Fat:

LUNCH	Calories:	Protein:	Carbs:	Fat:

DINNER	Calories:	Protein:	Carbs:	Fat:

SNACK 2	Calories:	Protein:	Carbs:	Fat:

PRE-WORKOUT SNACK	Calories:	Protein:	Carbs:	Fat:

POST-WORKOUT SNACK	Calories:	Protein:	Carbs:	Fat:

THURSDAY (DAY 32)

REST

NOTES

THURSDAY (DAY 32)

BREAKFAST	Calories:	Protein:	Carbs:	Fat:

SNACK 1	Calories:	Protein:	Carbs:	Fat:

LUNCH	Calories:	Protein:	Carbs:	Fat:

DINNER	Calories:	Protein:	Carbs:	Fat:

SNACK 2	Calories:	Protein:	Carbs:	Fat:

PRE-WORKOUT SNACK	Calories:	Protein:	Carbs:	Fat:

POST-WORKOUT SNACK	Calories:	Protein:	Carbs:	Fat:

FRIDAY (DAY 33)

5–10 min	WARM-UP *page 231*	

SET I		Reps / Time / Weight
9 reps	CHIN-UPS *page 216*	
12 reps	LUNGES EACH LEG *page 221*	
12 reps	PUSH-UPS *page 214*	
12 reps	HANGING LEG RAISES *page 218*	

SET 2		Reps / Time / Weight
8 reps	PULL-UPS *page 216*	
12	WOOD CHOPS *page 225*	
10 reps	DIAMOND PUSH-UPS *page 214*	
18 reps	SUPERMANS *page 219*	

SET 2		Reps / Time / Weight
8 reps	CHIN-UPS *page 216*	
14 reps	SQUATS *page 220*	
10 reps	PUSH-UPS *page 214*	
30 sec	SIDE PLANK EACH SIDE *page 224*	
10 min	CARDIO	
5–10 min	STRETCH *page 231*	

NOTES

FRIDAY (DAY 33)

BREAKFAST	Calories:	Protein:	Carbs:	Fat:

SNACK 1	Calories:	Protein:	Carbs:	Fat:

LUNCH	Calories:	Protein:	Carbs:	Fat:

DINNER	Calories:	Protein:	Carbs:	Fat:

SNACK 2	Calories:	Protein:	Carbs:	Fat:

PRE-WORKOUT SNACK	Calories:	Protein:	Carbs:	Fat:

POST-WORKOUT SNACK	Calories:	Protein:	Carbs:	Fat:

SATURDAY (DAY 34)

REST

NOTES

SATURDAY (DAY 34)

BREAKFAST	Calories:	Protein:	Carbs:	Fat:

SNACK I	Calories:	Protein:	Carbs:	Fat:

LUNCH	Calories:	Protein:	Carbs:	Fat:

DINNER	Calories:	Protein:	Carbs:	Fat:

SNACK 2	Calories:	Protein:	Carbs:	Fat:

PRE-WORKOUT SNACK	Calories:	Protein:	Carbs:	Fat:

POST-WORKOUT SNACK	Calories:	Protein:	Carbs:	Fat:

SUNDAY (DAY 35)

REST

NOTES

SUNDAY (DAY 35)

BREAKFAST	Calories:	Protein:	Carbs:	Fat:

SNACK 1	Calories:	Protein:	Carbs:	Fat:

LUNCH	Calories:	Protein:	Carbs:	Fat:

DINNER	Calories:	Protein:	Carbs:	Fat:

SNACK 2	Calories:	Protein:	Carbs:	Fat:

PRE-WORKOUT SNACK	Calories:	Protein:	Carbs:	Fat:

POST-WORKOUT SNACK	Calories:	Protein:	Carbs:	Fat:

MONDAY (DAY 36)

5–10 min	WARM-UP *page 231*	

SET 1		Reps / Time / Weight
10 reps	PULL-UPS *page 216*	
15 reps	SQUATS *page 220*	
14 reps	PUSH-UPS *page 214*	
14 reps	HANGING LEG RAISES *page 218*	

SET 2		Reps / Time / Weight
11 reps	CHIN-UPS *page 216*	
13 reps	LUNGES EACH LEG *page 221*	
15 reps	PUSH-UPS *page 214*	
1 min	PLANK *page 223*	

SET 3		Reps / Time / Weight
8 reps	PULL-UPS *page 216*	
12 reps	SQUATS *page 220*	
12 reps	NARROW PULL-UPS *page 216*	
24 reps	MASON TWISTS *page 226*	
5–10 min	STRETCH *page 231*	

NOTES

MONDAY (DAY 36)

BREAKFAST	Calories:	Protein:	Carbs:	Fat:

SNACK I	Calories:	Protein:	Carbs:	Fat:

LUNCH	Calories:	Protein:	Carbs:	Fat:

DINNER	Calories:	Protein:	Carbs:	Fat:

SNACK 2	Calories:	Protein:	Carbs:	Fat:

PRE-WORKOUT SNACK	Calories:	Protein:	Carbs:	Fat:

POST-WORKOUT SNACK	Calories:	Protein:	Carbs:	Fat:

TUESDAY (DAY 37)

REST

NOTES

TUESDAY (DAY 37)

BREAKFAST	Calories:	Protein:	Carbs:	Fat:

SNACK 1	Calories:	Protein:	Carbs:	Fat:

LUNCH	Calories:	Protein:	Carbs:	Fat:

DINNER	Calories:	Protein:	Carbs:	Fat:

SNACK 2	Calories:	Protein:	Carbs:	Fat:

PRE-WORKOUT SNACK	Calories:	Protein:	Carbs:	Fat:

POST-WORKOUT SNACK	Calories:	Protein:	Carbs:	Fat:

WEDNESDAY (DAY 38)

5–10 min	WARM-UP *page 231*	

SET 1		Reps / Time / Weight
11 reps	CHIN-UPS *page 216*	
13 reps	LUNGES EACH LEG *page 221*	
15 reps	PUSH-UPS *page 214*	
1 min	PLANK *page 223*	

SET 2		Reps / Time / Weight
10 reps	PULL-UPS *page 216*	
16 reps	SQUATS *page 220*	
12 reps	PUSH-UPS *page 214*	
15 reps	HANGING LEG RAISES *page 218*	

SET 3		Reps / Time / Weight
10 reps	CHIN-UPS *page 216*	
12 reps	LUNGES EACH LEG *page 221*	
10 reps	DIAMOND PUSH-UPS *page 214*	
24 reps	MASON TWISTS *page 226*	
5–10 min	STRETCH *page 231*	

NOTES

WEDNESDAY (DAY 38)

BREAKFAST	Calories:	Protein:	Carbs:	Fat:

SNACK 1	Calories:	Protein:	Carbs:	Fat:

LUNCH	Calories:	Protein:	Carbs:	Fat:

DINNER	Calories:	Protein:	Carbs:	Fat:

SNACK 2	Calories:	Protein:	Carbs:	Fat:

PRE-WORKOUT SNACK	Calories:	Protein:	Carbs:	Fat:

POST-WORKOUT SNACK	Calories:	Protein:	Carbs:	Fat:

THURSDAY (DAY 39)

REST

NOTES

THURSDAY (DAY 39)

BREAKFAST	Calories:	Protein:	Carbs:	Fat:

SNACK 1	Calories:	Protein:	Carbs:	Fat:

LUNCH	Calories:	Protein:	Carbs:	Fat:

DINNER	Calories:	Protein:	Carbs:	Fat:

SNACK 2	Calories:	Protein:	Carbs:	Fat:

PRE-WORKOUT SNACK	Calories:	Protein:	Carbs:	Fat:

POST-WORKOUT SNACK	Calories:	Protein:	Carbs:	Fat:

FRIDAY (DAY 40)

5–10 min	WARM-UP *page 231*	
SET 1		Reps / Time / Weight
10 reps	PULL-UPS *page 216*	
17 reps	SQUATS *page 220*	
16 reps	PUSH-UPS *page 214*	
15 reps	HANGING LEG RAISES *page 218*	
SET 2		Reps / Time / Weight
10 reps	BURPEES *page 227*	
30 sec	REST	
10 reps	DIAMOND PUSH-UPS *page 214*	
1 min	PLANK *page 223*	
SET 3		Reps / Time / Weight
9 reps	PULL-UPS *page 216*	
20 reps	SQUATS *page 220*	
12 reps	PUSH-UPS *page 214*	
15 reps	IN & OUTS *page 224*	
5–10 min	STRETCH *page 231*	

NOTES

FRIDAY (DAY 40)

BREAKFAST	Calories:	Protein:	Carbs:	Fat:

SNACK I	Calories:	Protein:	Carbs:	Fat:

LUNCH	Calories:	Protein:	Carbs:	Fat:

DINNER	Calories:	Protein:	Carbs:	Fat:

SNACK 2	Calories:	Protein:	Carbs:	Fat:

PRE-WORKOUT SNACK	Calories:	Protein:	Carbs:	Fat:

POST-WORKOUT SNACK	Calories:	Protein:	Carbs:	Fat:

SATURDAY (DAY 41)

REST

NOTES

SATURDAY (DAY 41)

BREAKFAST	Calories:	Protein:	Carbs:	Fat:

SNACK 1	Calories:	Protein:	Carbs:	Fat:

LUNCH	Calories:	Protein:	Carbs:	Fat:

DINNER	Calories:	Protein:	Carbs:	Fat:

SNACK 2	Calories:	Protein:	Carbs:	Fat:

PRE-WORKOUT SNACK	Calories:	Protein:	Carbs:	Fat:

POST-WORKOUT SNACK	Calories:	Protein:	Carbs:	Fat:

SUNDAY (DAY 42)

REST

NOTES

SUNDAY (DAY 42)

BREAKFAST	Calories:	Protein:	Carbs:	Fat:

SNACK 1	Calories:	Protein:	Carbs:	Fat:

LUNCH	Calories:	Protein:	Carbs:	Fat:

DINNER	Calories:	Protein:	Carbs:	Fat:

SNACK 2	Calories:	Protein:	Carbs:	Fat:

PRE-WORKOUT SNACK	Calories:	Protein:	Carbs:	Fat:

POST-WORKOUT SNACK	Calories:	Protein:	Carbs:	Fat:

MONDAY (DAY 43)

5–10 min	WARM-UP *page 231*	
SET I		Reps / Time / Weight
10 reps	PULL-UPS *page 216*	
18 reps	SQUATS *page 220*	
15 reps	PUSH-UPS *page 214*	
1 min	PLANK *page 223*	
SET 2		Reps / Time / Weight
11 reps	CHIN-UPS *page 216*	
13 reps	LUNGES EACH LEG *page 221*	
14 reps	NARROW PUSH-UPS *page 214*	
15 reps	HANGING LEG RAISES *page 218*	
SET 3		Reps / Time / Weight
10 reps	COMMANDO PULL-UPS *page 217*	
10 reps	SQUATS *page 220*	
12 reps	DIAMOND PUSH-UPS *page 214*	
22 reps	MOUNTAIN CLIMBERS *page 226*	
15 min	CARDIO	
5–10 min	STRETCH *page 231*	

NOTES

MONDAY (DAY 43)

BREAKFAST	Calories:	Protein:	Carbs:	Fat:

SNACK 1	Calories:	Protein:	Carbs:	Fat:

LUNCH	Calories:	Protein:	Carbs:	Fat:

DINNER	Calories:	Protein:	Carbs:	Fat:

SNACK 2	Calories:	Protein:	Carbs:	Fat:

PRE-WORKOUT SNACK	Calories:	Protein:	Carbs:	Fat:

POST-WORKOUT SNACK	Calories:	Protein:	Carbs:	Fat:

TUESDAY (DAY 44)

REST

NOTES

TUESDAY (DAY 44)

BREAKFAST	Calories:	Protein:	Carbs:	Fat:

SNACK I	Calories:	Protein:	Carbs:	Fat:

LUNCH	Calories:	Protein:	Carbs:	Fat:

DINNER	Calories:	Protein:	Carbs:	Fat:

SNACK 2	Calories:	Protein:	Carbs:	Fat:

PRE-WORKOUT SNACK	Calories:	Protein:	Carbs:	Fat:

POST-WORKOUT SNACK	Calories:	Protein:	Carbs:	Fat:

WEDNESDAY (DAY 45)

5–10 min	WARM-UP *page 231*	

SET 1		Reps / Time / Weight
12 reps	CHIN-UPS *page 216*	
10 reps	LUNGES WITH TWIST EACH LEG *page 222*	
8 reps	T PUSH-UPS *page 215*	
14 reps	AIR SQUATS *page 220*	

SET 2		Reps / Time / Weight
1 min	FOREARM PLANK *page 223*	
26 reps	MOUNTAIN CLIMBERS *page 226*	
12 reps	PUSH-UPS *page 214*	
10 reps	MOUNTAIN CLIMBERS *page 226*	
12 reps	SUPERMANS *page 219*	
1 min	FOREARM PLANK *page 223*	

SET 3		Reps / Time / Weight
10 reps	PULL-UPS *page 216*	
18 reps	SQUATS *page 220*	
15 min	CARDIO	
5–10 min	STRETCH *page 231*	

NOTES

WEDNESDAY (DAY 45)

BREAKFAST	Calories:	Protein:	Carbs:	Fat:

SNACK 1	Calories:	Protein:	Carbs:	Fat:

LUNCH	Calories:	Protein:	Carbs:	Fat:

DINNER	Calories:	Protein:	Carbs:	Fat:

SNACK 2	Calories:	Protein:	Carbs:	Fat:

PRE-WORKOUT SNACK	Calories:	Protein:	Carbs:	Fat:

POST-WORKOUT SNACK	Calories:	Protein:	Carbs:	Fat:

THURSDAY (DAY 46)

REST

NOTES

THURSDAY (DAY 46)

BREAKFAST	Calories:	Protein:	Carbs:	Fat:

SNACK 1	Calories:	Protein:	Carbs:	Fat:

LUNCH	Calories:	Protein:	Carbs:	Fat:

DINNER	Calories:	Protein:	Carbs:	Fat:

SNACK 2	Calories:	Protein:	Carbs:	Fat:

PRE-WORKOUT SNACK	Calories:	Protein:	Carbs:	Fat:

POST-WORKOUT SNACK	Calories:	Protein:	Carbs:	Fat:

FRIDAY (DAY 47)

5–10 min	WARM-UP *page 231*	

SET 1		Reps / Time / Weight
11 reps	PULL-UPS *page 216*	
20 reps	SQUATS WITH MEDICINE BALL *page 221*	
13 reps	DIAMOND PUSH-UPS *page 214*	
18 reps	HANGING LEG RAISES *page 218*	

SET 2		Reps / Time / Weight
70 sec	PLANK *page 223*	
10 reps	BURPEES *page 227*	
18 reps	MOUNTAIN CLIMBERS *page 226*	
30 reps	WOOD CHOPS *page 225*	

SET 3		Reps / Time / Weight
15 reps	CHIN-UPS *page 216*	
16 reps	HANGING LEG RAISES *page 218*	
10 reps	LUNGES WITH TWIST EACH LEG *page 222*	
12 reps	DIAMOND PUSH-UPS *page 214*	
15 min	CARDIO	
5–10 min	STRETCH *page 231*	

NOTES

FRIDAY (DAY 47)

BREAKFAST	Calories:	Protein:	Carbs:	Fat:

SNACK 1	Calories:	Protein:	Carbs:	Fat:

LUNCH	Calories:	Protein:	Carbs:	Fat:

DINNER	Calories:	Protein:	Carbs:	Fat:

SNACK 2	Calories:	Protein:	Carbs:	Fat:

PRE-WORKOUT SNACK	Calories:	Protein:	Carbs:	Fat:

POST-WORKOUT SNACK	Calories:	Protein:	Carbs:	Fat:

SATURDAY (DAY 48)

REST

NOTES

SATURDAY (DAY 48)

BREAKFAST	Calories:	Protein:	Carbs:	Fat:

SNACK I	Calories:	Protein:	Carbs:	Fat:

LUNCH	Calories:	Protein:	Carbs:	Fat:

DINNER	Calories:	Protein:	Carbs:	Fat:

SNACK 2	Calories:	Protein:	Carbs:	Fat:

PRE-WORKOUT SNACK	Calories:	Protein:	Carbs:	Fat:

POST-WORKOUT SNACK	Calories:	Protein:	Carbs:	Fat:

SUNDAY (DAY 49)

REST

NOTES

SUNDAY (DAY 49)

BREAKFAST	Calories:	Protein:	Carbs:	Fat:

SNACK 1	Calories:	Protein:	Carbs:	Fat:

LUNCH	Calories:	Protein:	Carbs:	Fat:

DINNER	Calories:	Protein:	Carbs:	Fat:

SNACK 2	Calories:	Protein:	Carbs:	Fat:

PRE-WORKOUT SNACK	Calories:	Protein:	Carbs:	Fat:

POST-WORKOUT SNACK	Calories:	Protein:	Carbs:	Fat:

MONDAY (DAY 50)

5–10 min	WARM-UP *page 231*	

SET 1		Reps / Time / Weight
12 reps	PULL-UPS *page 216*	
12 reps	SQUATS *page 220*	
8 reps	T PUSH-UPS EACH SIDE *page 215*	
75 sec	PLANK *page 223*	

SET 2		Reps / Time / Weight
12 reps	CHIN-UPS *page 216*	
16 reps	HANGING LEG RAISES *page 218*	
10 reps	BURPEES *page 227*	
8 reps	PUSH-UPS *page 214*	

SET 3		Reps / Time / Weight
10 reps	PULL-UPS *page 216*	
13 reps	LUNGES WITH TWIST EACH LEG *Page 222*	
30 reps	MOUNTAIN CLIMBERS *page 226*	
45 sec	SIDE PLANK EACH SIDE *page 224*	
12 reps	SUPERMANS *page 219*	
20 min	CARDIO	
5–10 min	STRETCH *page 231*	

NOTES

MONDAY (DAY 50)

BREAKFAST	Calories:	Protein:	Carbs:	Fat:

SNACK 1	Calories:	Protein:	Carbs:	Fat:

LUNCH	Calories:	Protein:	Carbs:	Fat:

DINNER	Calories:	Protein:	Carbs:	Fat:

SNACK 2	Calories:	Protein:	Carbs:	Fat:

PRE-WORKOUT SNACK	Calories:	Protein:	Carbs:	Fat:

POST-WORKOUT SNACK	Calories:	Protein:	Carbs:	Fat:

TUESDAY (DAY 51)

REST

NOTES

TUESDAY (DAY 51)

BREAKFAST	Calories:	Protein:	Carbs:	Fat:

SNACK 1	Calories:	Protein:	Carbs:	Fat:

LUNCH	Calories:	Protein:	Carbs:	Fat:

DINNER	Calories:	Protein:	Carbs:	Fat:

SNACK 2	Calories:	Protein:	Carbs:	Fat:

PRE-WORKOUT SNACK	Calories:	Protein:	Carbs:	Fat:

POST-WORKOUT SNACK	Calories:	Protein:	Carbs:	Fat:

WEDNESDAY (DAY 52)

5–10 min	WARM-UP *page 231*	

SET I		Reps / Time / Weight
TABATA INTERVALS (8 ROUNDS)		
20 sec	SQUATS *page 220*	
10 sec	REST BETWEEN ROUNDS	

SET2I		Reps / Time / Weight
TABATA INTERVALS (8 ROUNDS)		
20 sec	MOUNTAIN CLIMBERS *page 226*	
10 sec	REST BETWEEN ROUNDS	

SET 3		Reps / Time / Weight
TABATA INTERVALS (8 ROUNDS)		
20 sec	WOOD CHOPS (ALTERNATE SIDES) *page 225*	
10 sec	REST BETWEEN ROUNDS	

SET 4		Reps / Time / Weight
80 sec	PLANK *page 223*	
20 min	CARDIO	
5–10 min	STRETCH *page 231*	

NOTES

WEDNESDAY (DAY 52)

BREAKFAST	Calories:	Protein:	Carbs:	Fat:

SNACK 1	Calories:	Protein:	Carbs:	Fat:

LUNCH	Calories:	Protein:	Carbs:	Fat:

DINNER	Calories:	Protein:	Carbs:	Fat:

SNACK 2	Calories:	Protein:	Carbs:	Fat:

PRE-WORKOUT SNACK	Calories:	Protein:	Carbs:	Fat:

POST-WORKOUT SNACK	Calories:	Protein:	Carbs:	Fat:

THURSDAY (DAY 53)

REST

NOTES

THURSDAY (DAY 53)

BREAKFAST   Calories: Protein: Carbs: Fat:

SNACK I   Calories: Protein: Carbs: Fat:

LUNCH   Calories: Protein: Carbs: Fat:

DINNER   Calories: Protein: Carbs: Fat:

SNACK 2   Calories: Protein: Carbs: Fat:

PRE-WORKOUT SNACK   Calories: Protein: Carbs: Fat:

POST-WORKOUT SNACK   Calories: Protein: Carbs: Fat:

FRIDAY (DAY 54)

5–10 min	WARM-UP *page 231*	

SET 1		Reps / Time / Weight
14 reps	PULL-UPS *page 216*	
18 reps	AIR SQUATS *page 220*	
13 reps	DIAMOND PUSH-UPS *page 214*	
18 reps	HANGING LEG RAISES *page 218*	

SET 2		Reps / Time / Weight
70 sec	PLANK *page 223*	
15 reps	T PUSH-UPS EACH SIDE *page 215*	
26 reps	MOUNTAIN CLIMBERS *page 226*	
30 reps	WOOD CHOPS *page 225*	

SET 3		Reps / Time / Weight
10 reps	PULL-UPS *page 216*	
13 reps	LUNGES WITH TWIST EACH LEG *page 222*	
30 reps	MOUNTAIN CLIMBERS *page 226*	
45 sec	SIDE PLANK EACH SIDE *page 224*	
12 reps	SUPERMANS *page 219*	
20 min	CARDIO	
5–10 min	STRETCH *page 231*	

NOTES

FRIDAY (DAY 54)

BREAKFAST	Calories:	Protein:	Carbs:	Fat:

SNACK 1	Calories:	Protein:	Carbs:	Fat:

LUNCH	Calories:	Protein:	Carbs:	Fat:

DINNER	Calories:	Protein:	Carbs:	Fat:

SNACK 2	Calories:	Protein:	Carbs:	Fat:

PRE-WORKOUT SNACK	Calories:	Protein:	Carbs:	Fat:

POST-WORKOUT SNACK	Calories:	Protein:	Carbs:	Fat:

SATURDAY (DAY 55)

REST

NOTES

SATURDAY (DAY 55)

BREAKFAST	Calories:	Protein:	Carbs:	Fat:

SNACK 1	Calories:	Protein:	Carbs:	Fat:

LUNCH	Calories:	Protein:	Carbs:	Fat:

DINNER	Calories:	Protein:	Carbs:	Fat:

SNACK 2	Calories:	Protein:	Carbs:	Fat:

PRE-WORKOUT SNACK	Calories:	Protein:	Carbs:	Fat:

POST-WORKOUT SNACK	Calories:	Protein:	Carbs:	Fat:

SUNDAY (DAY 56)

REST

NOTES

SUNDAY (DAY 56)

BREAKFAST	Calories:	Protein:	Carbs:	Fat:

SNACK 1	Calories:	Protein:	Carbs:	Fat:

LUNCH	Calories:	Protein:	Carbs:	Fat:

DINNER	Calories:	Protein:	Carbs:	Fat:

SNACK 2	Calories:	Protein:	Carbs:	Fat:

PRE-WORKOUT SNACK	Calories:	Protein:	Carbs:	Fat:

POST-WORKOUT SNACK	Calories:	Protein:	Carbs:	Fat:

MONDAY (DAY 57)

5–10 min	WARM-UP *page 231*	

SET 2		Reps / Time / Weight
13 reps	PULL-UPS *page 216*	
24 reps	SQUATS WITH MEDICINE BALL *page 221*	
15 reps	PUSH-UPS *page 214*	
22 reps	IN & OUTS *page 224*	

SET 2		Reps / Time / Weight
80 sec	PLANK *page 223*	
15 reps	NARROW PUSH-UPS *page 214*	
26 reps	MOUNTAIN CLIMBERS *page 226*	
30 reps	WOOD CHOPS *page 225*	

SET 3		Reps / Time / Weight
15 reps	CHIN-UPS *page 216*	
16 reps	HANGING LEG RAISES *page 218*	
11 reps	LUNGES WITH TWIST EACH LEG P*age 222*	
12 reps	AIR SQUATS *page 220*	
20 min	CARDIO	
5–10 min	STRETCH *page 231*	

NOTES

MONDAY (DAY 57)

BREAKFAST	Calories:	Protein:	Carbs:	Fat:

SNACK 1	Calories:	Protein:	Carbs:	Fat:

LUNCH	Calories:	Protein:	Carbs:	Fat:

DINNER	Calories:	Protein:	Carbs:	Fat:

SNACK 2	Calories:	Protein:	Carbs:	Fat:

PRE-WORKOUT SNACK	Calories:	Protein:	Carbs:	Fat:

POST-WORKOUT SNACK	Calories:	Protein:	Carbs:	Fat:

TUESDAY (DAY 58)

REST

NOTES

TUESDAY (DAY 58)

BREAKFAST	Calories:	Protein:	Carbs:	Fat:

SNACK 1	Calories:	Protein:	Carbs:	Fat:

LUNCH	Calories:	Protein:	Carbs:	Fat:

DINNER	Calories:	Protein:	Carbs:	Fat:

SNACK 2	Calories:	Protein:	Carbs:	Fat:

PRE-WORKOUT SNACK	Calories:	Protein:	Carbs:	Fat:

POST-WORKOUT SNACK	Calories:	Protein:	Carbs:	Fat:

WEDNESDAY (DAY 59)

5–10 min	WARM-UP *page 231*	

SET I		Reps / Time / Weight
12 reps	CHIN-UPS *page 216*	
10 reps	LUNGES WITH TWIST EACH LEG *page 222*	
10 reps	PUSH-UPS *page 214*	
20 reps	SQUATS *page 220*	

SET 2		Reps / Time / Weight
1 min	FOREARM PLANK *page 223*	
20 reps	MOUNTAIN CLIMBERS *page 226*	
5 reps	T PUSH-UPS EACH SIDE *page 215*	
20 reps	REVERSE CRUNCHES *page 218*	
12 reps	SUPERMANS *page 219*	
45 sec	FLUTTER KICKS *page 228*	

SET 3		Reps / Time / Weight
10 reps	PULL-UPS *page 216*	
24 reps	WOOD CHOPS *page 225*	
20 min	CARDIO	
5–10 min	STRETCH *page 231*	

NOTES

WEDNESDAY (DAY 59)

BREAKFAST	Calories:	Protein:	Carbs:	Fat:

SNACK 1	Calories:	Protein:	Carbs:	Fat:

LUNCH	Calories:	Protein:	Carbs:	Fat:

DINNER	Calories:	Protein:	Carbs:	Fat:

SNACK 2	Calories:	Protein:	Carbs:	Fat:

PRE-WORKOUT SNACK	Calories:	Protein:	Carbs:	Fat:

POST-WORKOUT SNACK	Calories:	Protein:	Carbs:	Fat:

THURSDAY (DAY 60)

REST

NOTES

THURSDAY (DAY 60)

BREAKFAST	Calories:	Protein:	Carbs:	Fat:

SNACK 1	Calories:	Protein:	Carbs:	Fat:

LUNCH	Calories:	Protein:	Carbs:	Fat:

DINNER	Calories:	Protein:	Carbs:	Fat:

SNACK 2	Calories:	Protein:	Carbs:	Fat:

PRE-WORKOUT SNACK	Calories:	Protein:	Carbs:	Fat:

POST-WORKOUT SNACK	Calories:	Protein:	Carbs:	Fat:

FRIDAY (DAY 61)

5–10 min	WARM-UP *page 231*	

SET I		Reps / Time / Weight
12 reps	COMMANDO PULL-UPS *page 217*	
16 reps	HANGING LEG RAISES *page 218*	
6 reps	CHIN-UPS *page 216*	
8 reps	HANGING LEG RAISES *page 218*	

SET 2		Reps / Time / Weight
14 reps	SQUATS *page 220*	
12 reps	LUNGES *page 221*	

SET 3		Reps / Time / Weight
15 reps	AIR SQUATS *page 220*	
7 reps	LUNGES WITH TWIST EACH LEG *page 222*	

SET 4		Reps / Time / Weight
1 min	PLANK *page 223*	
26 reps	MOUNTAIN CLIMBERS *page 226*	
12 reps	MEDICINE BALL PUSH-UPS *page 215*	
20 min	CARDIO	
5–10 min	STRETCH *page 231*	

NOTES

FRIDAY (DAY 61)

BREAKFAST	Calories:	Protein:	Carbs:	Fat:

SNACK 1	Calories:	Protein:	Carbs:	Fat:

LUNCH	Calories:	Protein:	Carbs:	Fat:

DINNER	Calories:	Protein:	Carbs:	Fat:

SNACK 2	Calories:	Protein:	Carbs:	Fat:

PRE-WORKOUT SNACK	Calories:	Protein:	Carbs:	Fat:

POST-WORKOUT SNACK	Calories:	Protein:	Carbs:	Fat:

SATURDAY (DAY 62)

REST

NOTES

SATURDAY (DAY 62)

BREAKFAST	Calories:	Protein:	Carbs:	Fat:

SNACK 1	Calories:	Protein:	Carbs:	Fat:

LUNCH	Calories:	Protein:	Carbs:	Fat:

DINNER	Calories:	Protein:	Carbs:	Fat:

SNACK 2	Calories:	Protein:	Carbs:	Fat:

PRE-WORKOUT SNACK	Calories:	Protein:	Carbs:	Fat:

POST-WORKOUT SNACK	Calories:	Protein:	Carbs:	Fat:

SUNDAY (DAY 63)

REST

NOTES

SUNDAY (DAY 63)

BREAKFAST	Calories:	Protein:	Carbs:	Fat:

SNACK 1	Calories:	Protein:	Carbs:	Fat:

LUNCH	Calories:	Protein:	Carbs:	Fat:

DINNER	Calories:	Protein:	Carbs:	Fat:

SNACK 2	Calories:	Protein:	Carbs:	Fat:

PRE-WORKOUT SNACK	Calories:	Protein:	Carbs:	Fat:

POST-WORKOUT SNACK	Calories:	Protein:	Carbs:	Fat:

MONDAY (DAY 64)

5–10 min	WARM-UP *page 231*	

SET I		Reps / Time / Weight
TABATA INTERVALS (8 ROUNDS)		
20 sec	AIR SQUATS *page 220*	
10 sec	REST BETWEEN ROUNDS	

SET 2		Reps / Time / Weight
TABATA INTERVALS (8 ROUNDS)		
20 sec	MOUNTAIN CLIMBERS *page 226*	
10 sec	REST BETWEEN ROUNDS	

SET 3		Reps / Time / Weight
TABATA INTERVALS (8 ROUNDS)		
20 sec	JUMPING JACKS *page 227*	
10 sec	REST	
20 sec	BUTT KICKS *page 229*	
10 sec	REST	
20 sec	WOOD CHOPS *page 225*	
10 sec	REST	
20 sec	HIGH KNEES *page 230*	
10 sec	REST	
REPEAT		

SET 4		Reps / Time / Weight
80 sec	PLANK *page 223*	
20 min	CARDIO	
5–10 min	STRETCH *page 231*	
NOTES		

MONDAY (DAY 64)

BREAKFAST	Calories:	Protein:	Carbs:	Fat:

SNACK 1	Calories:	Protein:	Carbs:	Fat:

LUNCH	Calories:	Protein:	Carbs:	Fat:

DINNER	Calories:	Protein:	Carbs:	Fat:

SNACK 2	Calories:	Protein:	Carbs:	Fat:

PRE-WORKOUT SNACK	Calories:	Protein:	Carbs:	Fat:

POST-WORKOUT SNACK	Calories:	Protein:	Carbs:	Fat:

TUESDAY (DAY 65)

REST

NOTES

TUESDAY (DAY 65)

BREAKFAST	Calories:	Protein:	Carbs:	Fat:

SNACK I	Calories:	Protein:	Carbs:	Fat:

LUNCH	Calories:	Protein:	Carbs:	Fat:

DINNER	Calories:	Protein:	Carbs:	Fat:

SNACK 2	Calories:	Protein:	Carbs:	Fat:

PRE-WORKOUT SNACK	Calories:	Protein:	Carbs:	Fat:

POST-WORKOUT SNACK	Calories:	Protein:	Carbs:	Fat:

WEDNESDAY (DAY 66)

5–10 min	WARM-UP *page 231*	

SET 1		Reps / Time / Weight
14 reps	PULL-UPS *page 216*	
26 reps	SQUATS WITH MEDICINE BALL *page 221*	
18 reps	PUSH-UPS *page 214*	
75 sec	PLANK *page 223*	

SET 2		Reps / Time / Weight
15 reps	COMMANDO PULL-UPS *page 217*	
16 reps	HANGING LEG RAISES *page 218*	
30 reps	WOOD CHOPS *page 225*	
12 reps	MEDICINE BALL PUSH-UPS *page 214*	

SET 3		Reps / Time / Weight
14 reps	BURPEES *page 227*	
13 reps	LUNGES WITH TWIST EACH LEG *page 222*	
30 reps	MOUNTAIN CLIMBERS *page 226*	
45 sec	FLUTTER KICKS *page 228*	
12 reps	SUPERMANS *page 219*	
20 min	CARDIO	
5–10 min	STRETCH *page 231*	

NOTES

WEDNESDAY (DAY 66)

BREAKFAST	Calories:	Protein:	Carbs:	Fat:

SNACK 1	Calories:	Protein:	Carbs:	Fat:

LUNCH	Calories:	Protein:	Carbs:	Fat:

DINNER	Calories:	Protein:	Carbs:	Fat:

SNACK 2	Calories:	Protein:	Carbs:	Fat:

PRE-WORKOUT SNACK	Calories:	Protein:	Carbs:	Fat:

POST-WORKOUT SNACK	Calories:	Protein:	Carbs:	Fat:

THURSDAY (DAY 67)

REST

NOTES

THURSDAY (DAY 67)

BREAKFAST	Calories:	Protein:	Carbs:	Fat:

SNACK I	Calories:	Protein:	Carbs:	Fat:

LUNCH	Calories:	Protein:	Carbs:	Fat:

DINNER	Calories:	Protein:	Carbs:	Fat:

SNACK 2	Calories:	Protein:	Carbs:	Fat:

PRE-WORKOUT SNACK	Calories:	Protein:	Carbs:	Fat:

POST-WORKOUT SNACK	Calories:	Protein:	Carbs:	Fat:

FRIDAY (DAY 68)

5–10 min	WARM-UP *page 231*	

SET 1		Reps / Time / Weight
20 reps	SQUATS WITH MEDICINE BALL *page 221*	
6 reps	LUNGES WITH TWIST EACH LEG *page 222*	

SET 2		Reps / Time / Weight
12 reps	PULL-UPS *page 216*	
16 reps	HANGING LEG RAISES *page 218*	
5 reps	CHIN-UPS *page 216*	
10 reps	HANGING LEG RAISES *page 218*	

SET 3		Reps / Time / Weight
15 reps	AIR SQUATS *page 220*	
7 reps	LUNGES WITH TWIST EACH LEG *page 222*	

SET 3		Reps / Time / Weight
1 min	PLANK *page 223*	
30 reps	MOUNTAIN CLIMBERS *page 226*	
12 reps	MEDICINE BALL PUSH-UPS *page 214*	
12 reps	SUPERMANS *page 219*	
20 min	CARDIO	
5–10 min	STRETCH *page 231*	

NOTES

FRIDAY (DAY 68)

BREAKFAST	Calories:	Protein:	Carbs:	Fat:

SNACK 1	Calories:	Protein:	Carbs:	Fat:

LUNCH	Calories:	Protein:	Carbs:	Fat:

DINNER	Calories:	Protein:	Carbs:	Fat:

SNACK 2	Calories:	Protein:	Carbs:	Fat:

PRE-WORKOUT SNACK	Calories:	Protein:	Carbs:	Fat:

POST-WORKOUT SNACK	Calories:	Protein:	Carbs:	Fat:

SATURDAY (DAY 69)

REST

NOTES

SATURDAY (DAY 69)

BREAKFAST	Calories:	Protein:	Carbs:	Fat:

SNACK I	Calories:	Protein:	Carbs:	Fat:

LUNCH	Calories:	Protein:	Carbs:	Fat:

DINNER	Calories:	Protein:	Carbs:	Fat:

SNACK 2	Calories:	Protein:	Carbs:	Fat:

PRE-WORKOUT SNACK	Calories:	Protein:	Carbs:	Fat:

POST-WORKOUT SNACK	Calories:	Protein:	Carbs:	Fat:

SUNDAY (DAY 70)

REST

NOTES

SUNDAY (DAY 70)

BREAKFAST	Calories:	Protein:	Carbs:	Fat:

SNACK I	Calories:	Protein:	Carbs:	Fat:

LUNCH	Calories:	Protein:	Carbs:	Fat:

DINNER	Calories:	Protein:	Carbs:	Fat:

SNACK 2	Calories:	Protein:	Carbs:	Fat:

PRE-WORKOUT SNACK	Calories:	Protein:	Carbs:	Fat:

POST-WORKOUT SNACK	Calories:	Protein:	Carbs:	Fat:

MONDAY (DAY 71)

5–10 min	WARM-UP *page 231*	

SET 1		Reps / Time / Weight
10 reps	PUSH-UPS *page 214*	
10 reps	SQUATS *page 220*	

SET 2		Reps / Time / Weight
15 reps	PUSH-UPS *page 214*	
15 reps	SQUATS *page 220*	

SET 3		Reps / Time / Weight
10 reps	PUSH-UPS *page 214*	
10 reps	SQUATS *page 220*	

SET 4		Reps / Time / Weight
5 reps	PUSH-UPS *page 214*	
5 reps	SQUATS *page 220*	
5–10 min	STRETCH *page 231*	

NOTES

MONDAY (DAY 71)

BREAKFAST	Calories:	Protein:	Carbs:	Fat:

SNACK 1	Calories:	Protein:	Carbs:	Fat:

LUNCH	Calories:	Protein:	Carbs:	Fat:

DINNER	Calories:	Protein:	Carbs:	Fat:

SNACK 2	Calories:	Protein:	Carbs:	Fat:

PRE-WORKOUT SNACK	Calories:	Protein:	Carbs:	Fat:

POST-WORKOUT SNACK	Calories:	Protein:	Carbs:	Fat:

TUESDAY (DAY 72)

REST

NOTES

TUESDAY (DAY 72)

BREAKFAST	Calories:	Protein:	Carbs:	Fat:

SNACK 1	Calories:	Protein:	Carbs:	Fat:

LUNCH	Calories:	Protein:	Carbs:	Fat:

DINNER	Calories:	Protein:	Carbs:	Fat:

SNACK 2	Calories:	Protein:	Carbs:	Fat:

PRE-WORKOUT SNACK	Calories:	Protein:	Carbs:	Fat:

POST-WORKOUT SNACK	Calories:	Protein:	Carbs:	Fat:

WEDNESDAY (DAY 73)

5–10 min	WARM-UP *page 231*	

SET 1		Reps / Time / Weight
5 reps	LUNGES EACH SIDE *page 221*	
5 reps	PULL-UPS *page 216*	

SET 2		Reps / Time / Weight
8 reps	LUNGES EACH SIDE *page 221*	
8 reps	CHIN-UPS *page 216*	

SET 3		Reps / Time / Weight
10 reps	LUNGES EACH SIDE *page 221*	
10 reps	NARROW PULL-UPS *page 216*	

SET 4		Reps / Time / Weight
5 reps	LUNGES EACH SIDE *page 221*	
5 reps	PULL-UPS *page 216*	
5–10 min	STRETCH *page 231*	

NOTES

WEDNESDAY (DAY 73)

BREAKFAST	Calories:	Protein:	Carbs:	Fat:

SNACK 1	Calories:	Protein:	Carbs:	Fat:

LUNCH	Calories:	Protein:	Carbs:	Fat:

DINNER	Calories:	Protein:	Carbs:	Fat:

SNACK 2	Calories:	Protein:	Carbs:	Fat:

PRE-WORKOUT SNACK	Calories:	Protein:	Carbs:	Fat:

POST-WORKOUT SNACK	Calories:	Protein:	Carbs:	Fat:

THURSDAY (DAY 74)

REST

NOTES

THURSDAY (DAY 74)

BREAKFAST	Calories:	Protein:	Carbs:	Fat:

SNACK 1	Calories:	Protein:	Carbs:	Fat:

LUNCH	Calories:	Protein:	Carbs:	Fat:

DINNER	Calories:	Protein:	Carbs:	Fat:

SNACK 2	Calories:	Protein:	Carbs:	Fat:

PRE-WORKOUT SNACK	Calories:	Protein:	Carbs:	Fat:

POST-WORKOUT SNACK	Calories:	Protein:	Carbs:	Fat:

FRIDAY (DAY 75)		
5–10 min	WARM-UP *page 231*	
SET I		Reps / Time / Weight
1 min	PLANK *page 223*	
20 reps	FLUTTER KICKS *page 228*	
SET 2		Reps / Time / Weight
30 sec	SIDE PLANK EACH SIDE *page 224*	
10 reps	IN & OUTS *page 224*	
SET 2		Reps / Time / Weight
1 min	PLANK *page 223*	
20 reps	FLUTTER KICKS *page 228*	
SET 3		Reps / Time / Weight
30 sec	SIDE PLANK EACH SIDE *page 224*	
20 reps	MASON TWISTS *page 226*	
5–10 min	STRETCH *page 231*	

NOTES

FRIDAY (DAY 75)

BREAKFAST	Calories:	Protein:	Carbs:	Fat:

SNACK I	Calories:	Protein:	Carbs:	Fat:

LUNCH	Calories:	Protein:	Carbs:	Fat:

DINNER	Calories:	Protein:	Carbs:	Fat:

SNACK 2	Calories:	Protein:	Carbs:	Fat:

PRE-WORKOUT SNACK	Calories:	Protein:	Carbs:	Fat:

POST-WORKOUT SNACK	Calories:	Protein:	Carbs:	Fat:

SATURDAY (DAY 76)

REST

NOTES

SATURDAY (DAY 76)

BREAKFAST	Calories:	Protein:	Carbs:	Fat:

SNACK 1	Calories:	Protein:	Carbs:	Fat:

LUNCH	Calories:	Protein:	Carbs:	Fat:

DINNER	Calories:	Protein:	Carbs:	Fat:

SNACK 2	Calories:	Protein:	Carbs:	Fat:

PRE-WORKOUT SNACK	Calories:	Protein:	Carbs:	Fat:

POST-WORKOUT SNACK	Calories:	Protein:	Carbs:	Fat:

SUNDAY (DAY 77)

REST

NOTES

SUNDAY (DAY 77)

BREAKFAST	Calories:	Protein:	Carbs:	Fat:

SNACK 1	Calories:	Protein:	Carbs:	Fat:

LUNCH	Calories:	Protein:	Carbs:	Fat:

DINNER	Calories:	Protein:	Carbs:	Fat:

SNACK 2	Calories:	Protein:	Carbs:	Fat:

PRE-WORKOUT SNACK	Calories:	Protein:	Carbs:	Fat:

POST-WORKOUT SNACK	Calories:	Protein:	Carbs:	Fat:

MONDAY (DAY 78)		
5–10 min	WARM-UP *page 231*	
SET I		Reps / Time / Weight
20 reps	AIR SQUATS *page 220*	
20 reps	MARCHING TWISTS *page 225*	
SET 2		Reps / Time / Weight
10 reps	JUMPING LUNGES EACH SIDE *page 222*	
10 reps	INCHWORMS *page 230*	
SET 3		Reps / Time / Weight
15 reps	AIR SQUATS *page 220*	
15 reps	MARCHING TWISTS *page 225*	
SET 4		Reps / Time / Weight
10 reps	JUMPING LUNGES EACH SIDE *page 222*	
10 reps	INCHWORMS *page 230*	
20 min	CARDIO	
5–10 min	STRETCH *page 231*	

NOTES

MONDAY (DAY 78)

BREAKFAST	Calories:	Protein:	Carbs:	Fat:

SNACK 1	Calories:	Protein:	Carbs:	Fat:

LUNCH	Calories:	Protein:	Carbs:	Fat:

DINNER	Calories:	Protein:	Carbs:	Fat:

SNACK 2	Calories:	Protein:	Carbs:	Fat:

PRE-WORKOUT SNACK	Calories:	Protein:	Carbs:	Fat:

POST-WORKOUT SNACK	Calories:	Protein:	Carbs:	Fat:

TUESDAY (DAY 79)

REST

NOTES

TUESDAY (DAY 79)

BREAKFAST	Calories:	Protein:	Carbs:	Fat:

SNACK 1	Calories:	Protein:	Carbs:	Fat:

LUNCH	Calories:	Protein:	Carbs:	Fat:

DINNER	Calories:	Protein:	Carbs:	Fat:

SNACK 2	Calories:	Protein:	Carbs:	Fat:

PRE-WORKOUT SNACK	Calories:	Protein:	Carbs:	Fat:

POST-WORKOUT SNACK	Calories:	Protein:	Carbs:	Fat:

WEDNESDAY (DAY 80)

5–10 min	WARM-UP *page 231*	

SET 1		Reps / Time / Weight
20 reps	BURPEES *page 227*	
20 reps	REVERSE CRUNCHES *page 218*	
20 reps	HIP RAISES *page 229*	

SET 2		Reps / Time / Weight
15 reps	BURPEES *page 227*	
15 reps	IN & OUTS *page 224*	

SET 3		Reps / Time / Weight
10 reps	BURPEES *page 227*	
10 reps	JUMPING LUNGES EACH SIDE *page 222*	

SET 4		Reps / Time / Weight
8 reps	BURPEES *page 227*	
8 reps	IN & OUTS *page 224*	
20 min	CARDIO	
5–10 min	STRETCH *page 231*	

NOTES

WEDNESDAY (DAY 80)

BREAKFAST	Calories:	Protein:	Carbs:	Fat:

SNACK 1	Calories:	Protein:	Carbs:	Fat:

LUNCH	Calories:	Protein:	Carbs:	Fat:

DINNER	Calories:	Protein:	Carbs:	Fat:

SNACK 2	Calories:	Protein:	Carbs:	Fat:

PRE-WORKOUT SNACK	Calories:	Protein:	Carbs:	Fat:

POST-WORKOUT SNACK	Calories:	Protein:	Carbs:	Fat:

THURSDAY (DAY 81)

REST

NOTES

THURSDAY (DAY 81)

BREAKFAST	Calories:	Protein:	Carbs:	Fat:

SNACK 1	Calories:	Protein:	Carbs:	Fat:

LUNCH	Calories:	Protein:	Carbs:	Fat:

DINNER	Calories:	Protein:	Carbs:	Fat:

SNACK 2	Calories:	Protein:	Carbs:	Fat:

PRE-WORKOUT SNACK	Calories:	Protein:	Carbs:	Fat:

POST-WORKOUT SNACK	Calories:	Protein:	Carbs:	Fat:

FRIDAY (DAY 82)

5–10 min	WARM-UP *page 231*	

SET I		Reps / Time / Weight
TABATA INTERVALS (8 ROUNDS)		
20 sec	MOUNTAIN CLIMBERS *page 226*	
10 sec	REST BETWEEN ROUNDS	

SET 2		Reps / Time / Weight
TABATA INTERVALS (8 ROUNDS)		
20 sec	JUMPING LUNGES EACH SIDE *page 222*	
10 sec	REST BETWEEN ROUNDS	

SET 3		Reps / Time / Weight
TABATA INTERVALS (8 ROUNDS)		
20 sec	JUMPING JACKS *page 227*	
10 sec	REST	
20 sec	BUTT KICKS *page 229*	
10 sec	REST	
REPEAT 3 TIMES		

SET 4		Reps / Time / Weight
TABATA INTERVALS (8 ROUNDS)		
20 sec	WOOD CHOPS *page 225*	
10 sec	REST	
20 sec	HIGH KNEES *page 230*	
10 sec	REST	
REPEAT 3 TIMES		
20 min	CARDIO	
5–10 min	STRETCH *page 231*	

FRIDAY (DAY 82)

BREAKFAST	Calories:	Protein:	Carbs:	Fat:

SNACK 1	Calories:	Protein:	Carbs:	Fat:

LUNCH	Calories:	Protein:	Carbs:	Fat:

DINNER	Calories:	Protein:	Carbs:	Fat:

SNACK 2	Calories:	Protein:	Carbs:	Fat:

PRE-WORKOUT SNACK	Calories:	Protein:	Carbs:	Fat:

POST-WORKOUT SNACK	Calories:	Protein:	Carbs:	Fat:

SATURDAY (DAY 83)

REST

NOTES

SATURDAY (DAY 83)

BREAKFAST	Calories:	Protein:	Carbs:	Fat:

SNACK I	Calories:	Protein:	Carbs:	Fat:

LUNCH	Calories:	Protein:	Carbs:	Fat:

DINNER	Calories:	Protein:	Carbs:	Fat:

SNACK 2	Calories:	Protein:	Carbs:	Fat:

PRE-WORKOUT SNACK	Calories:	Protein:	Carbs:	Fat:

POST-WORKOUT SNACK	Calories:	Protein:	Carbs:	Fat:

SUNDAY (DAY 84)

REST

NOTES

SUNDAY (DAY 84)

BREAKFAST	Calories:	Protein:	Carbs:	Fat:

SNACK 1	Calories:	Protein:	Carbs:	Fat:

LUNCH	Calories:	Protein:	Carbs:	Fat:

DINNER	Calories:	Protein:	Carbs:	Fat:

SNACK 2	Calories:	Protein:	Carbs:	Fat:

PRE-WORKOUT SNACK	Calories:	Protein:	Carbs:	Fat:

POST-WORKOUT SNACK	Calories:	Protein:	Carbs:	Fat:

MONDAY (DAY 85)

5–10 min	WARM-UP *page 231*	
SET 1		Reps / Time / Weight
20 reps	PUSH-UPS *page 214*	
20 reps	IN & OUTS *page 224*	
SET 2		Reps / Time / Weight
20 reps	DIAMOND PUSH-UPS *page 214*	
20 reps	SUPERMANS *page 219*	
SET 3		Reps / Time / Weight
10 reps	T PUSH-UPS EACH SIDE *page 215*	
20 reps	HIP RAISES *page 229*	
SET 4		Reps / Time / Weight
20 reps	PUSH-UPS *page 214*	
20 reps	REVERSE CRUNCHES *page 218*	
20 min	CARDIO	
5–10 min	STRETCH *page 231*	

NOTES

MONDAY (DAY 85)

BREAKFAST	Calories:	Protein:	Carbs:	Fat:

SNACK 1	Calories:	Protein:	Carbs:	Fat:

LUNCH	Calories:	Protein:	Carbs:	Fat:

DINNER	Calories:	Protein:	Carbs:	Fat:

SNACK 2	Calories:	Protein:	Carbs:	Fat:

PRE-WORKOUT SNACK	Calories:	Protein:	Carbs:	Fat:

POST-WORKOUT SNACK	Calories:	Protein:	Carbs:	Fat:

TUESDAY (DAY 86)

REST

NOTES

TUESDAY (DAY 86)

BREAKFAST	Calories:	Protein:	Carbs:	Fat:

SNACK I	Calories:	Protein:	Carbs:	Fat:

LUNCH	Calories:	Protein:	Carbs:	Fat:

DINNER	Calories:	Protein:	Carbs:	Fat:

SNACK 2	Calories:	Protein:	Carbs:	Fat:

PRE-WORKOUT SNACK	Calories:	Protein:	Carbs:	Fat:

POST-WORKOUT SNACK	Calories:	Protein:	Carbs:	Fat:

WEDNESDAY (DAY 87)

5–10 min	WARM-UP *page 231*	
SET 1		Reps / Time / Weight
TABATA INTERVALS (8 ROUNDS)		
20 sec	LUNGES *page 221*	
10 sec	REST BETWEEN ROUNDS	
SET 2		Reps / Time / Weight
TABATA INTERVALS (8 ROUNDS)		
20 sec	PUSH-UPS *page 214*	
10 sec	REST BETWEEN ROUNDS	
SET 3		Reps / Time / Weight
TABATA INTERVALS (8 ROUNDS)		
20 sec	JUMPING JACKS *page 227*	
10 sec	REST	
SET 4		Reps / Time / Weight
TABATA INTERVALS (8 ROUNDS)		
20 sec	SQUATS *page 220*	
10 sec	REST	
SET 5		Reps / Time / Weight
20 min	CARDIO	
5–10 min	STRETCH *page 231*	

NOTES

WEDNESDAY (DAY 87)

BREAKFAST	Calories:	Protein:	Carbs:	Fat:

SNACK 1	Calories:	Protein:	Carbs:	Fat:

LUNCH	Calories:	Protein:	Carbs:	Fat:

DINNER	Calories:	Protein:	Carbs:	Fat:

SNACK 2	Calories:	Protein:	Carbs:	Fat:

PRE-WORKOUT SNACK	Calories:	Protein:	Carbs:	Fat:

POST-WORKOUT SNACK	Calories:	Protein:	Carbs:	Fat:

THURSDAY (DAY 88)

REST

NOTES

THURSDAY (DAY 88)

BREAKFAST	Calories:	Protein:	Carbs:	Fat:

SNACK 1	Calories:	Protein:	Carbs:	Fat:

LUNCH	Calories:	Protein:	Carbs:	Fat:

DINNER	Calories:	Protein:	Carbs:	Fat:

SNACK 2	Calories:	Protein:	Carbs:	Fat:

PRE-WORKOUT SNACK	Calories:	Protein:	Carbs:	Fat:

POST-WORKOUT SNACK	Calories:	Protein:	Carbs:	Fat:

FRIDAY (DAY 89)		
5–10 min	WARM-UP *page 231*	
SET I		Reps / Time / Weight
20 reps	BICYCLE CRUNCHES *page 219*	
90 sec	PLANK *page 223*	
SET 2		Reps / Time / Weight
20 reps	MASON TWISTS *page 226*	
80 sec	PLANK *page 223*	
SET 3		Reps / Time / Weight
20 reps	HIP RAISES *page 229*	
70 sec	PLANK *page 223*	
SET 4		Reps / Time / Weight
20 reps	MOUNTAIN CLIMBERS *page 226*	
1 min	PLANK *page 223*	
20 min	CARDIO	
5–10 min	STRETCH *page 231*	

NOTES

FRIDAY (DAY 89)

BREAKFAST	Calories:	Protein:	Carbs:	Fat:

SNACK 1	Calories:	Protein:	Carbs:	Fat:

LUNCH	Calories:	Protein:	Carbs:	Fat:

DINNER	Calories:	Protein:	Carbs:	Fat:

SNACK 2	Calories:	Protein:	Carbs:	Fat:

PRE-WORKOUT SNACK	Calories:	Protein:	Carbs:	Fat:

POST-WORKOUT SNACK	Calories:	Protein:	Carbs:	Fat:

SATURDAY (DAY 90)

REST

NOTES

SATURDAY (DAY 90)

BREAKFAST	Calories:	Protein:	Carbs:	Fat:

SNACK 1	Calories:	Protein:	Carbs:	Fat:

LUNCH	Calories:	Protein:	Carbs:	Fat:

DINNER	Calories:	Protein:	Carbs:	Fat:

SNACK 2	Calories:	Protein:	Carbs:	Fat:

PRE-WORKOUT SNACK	Calories:	Protein:	Carbs:	Fat:

POST-WORKOUT SNACK	Calories:	Protein:	Carbs:	Fat:

AFTER THE JOURNAL

Congratulations on completing *The Gym-Free Journal* program. I sincerely hope the exercises and workouts helped you meet your short-term fitness goals. So, now it's time to think about what your long-term goals are and how you can achieve them—and how the foundation that you've built with *The Gym-Free Journal* can help.

As I shared way back on page 9, "Your success depends on building a sustainable routine that's familiar, comfortable and repeatable." And now that you've done that hard work, you can adjust your thinking to the broad view of continuing to reach your fitness goals while developing a healthy, active lifestyle.

Lifelong fitness needs to be viewed as a relationship; there will be ups and downs along the way that you'll have to learn how to roll with in order to adapt and grow as you age, your activities change, and your real-life situations require. Depending on the type of year-round weather your region has and the type of sport-specific physical activity you participate in, your long-term goal should be to schedule one to three "peak seasons" throughout the year, during which you'll target optimal training and nutrition to prepare for an event like a marathon, a season like your company's softball team, or a vacation at the beach. To that end, follow the program in this book, focusing on high intensity and developing your strength or speed. Consider the months in between these peak training times as your off-season, when you'll maintain your fitness with relatively easy workouts at lower intensity and adapt the exercise and nutrition to suit your lifestyle for mental and physical recovery and refocusing. My advice is to run two to three days per week at a medium pace and perform two to three sets of bodyweight exercises twice a week to stay limber and fit.

Now, if you're looking for a new challenge, I've got you covered! Whether you'd like to tackle an obstacle race or mud run, complete a triathlon, run a 5K to a marathon, get your body in tip-top ripped shape, or develop elite athletic speed, strength and endurance through Functional Cross Training (FXT), I've written books that cover all of those topics and more! Visit me at www.7weekstofitness.com, where you can download samples of each of my books, test out the programs, register for more-advanced programs and mobile apps, and find just about everything you need to get—and stay—fit!

PART 3: THE EXERCISES

PUSH-UP

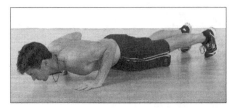

1 Place your hands on the ground approximately shoulder-width apart, making sure your fingers point straight ahead and your arms are straight but your elbows not locked. Step your feet back until your body forms a straight line from head to feet. Your feet should be about 6 inches apart with the weight in the balls of your feet. Engage your core to keep your spine from sagging; don't sink into your shoulders. **2** Inhale as you lower your torso to the ground and focus on keeping your elbows as close to your sides as possible, stopping when your elbows are at a 90° angle or your chest is 1–2 inches from the floor. **3** Using your shoulders, chest and triceps, exhale and push your torso back up to starting position.

DIAMOND PUSH-UP

This version targets the triceps more than standard push-ups do.

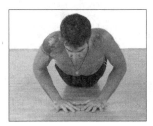

Place your hands directly under your chest with the thumb and forefinger of each hand touching to form a "diamond."

NARROW VARIATION: This version also targets the triceps more than standard push-ups do. Here, your hands are 6–10 inches apart, but not making the diamond shape.

MEDICINE BALL PUSH-UP

Medicine ball push-ups require you to use a host of different supporting muscles throughout your upper body and core to stay stable while you complete the movement.

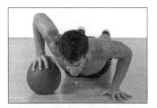

1 Assume a push-up position but place a medicine ball under one hand while keeping the other hand flat on the floor. Engage your core to keep your spine erect and keep your body in a straight line from head to toe.   **2** Inhale as you lower your upper body toward the floor, stopping when your chest is about 1 inch above the medicine ball.   **3** Exhale and push off the floor using your arms, chest, back and core and return to starting position. Place both hands on the floor and walk your hands to the left or right to place your other hand on top of the ball. Repeat until all reps are complete.

T PUSH-UP

This exercise gets its name from the ending position when your body forms a "T."

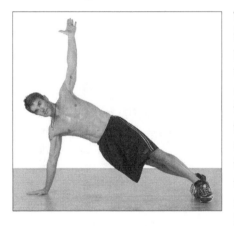

1 Assume a standard push-up position (page 214).   **2** Inhale as you lower your torso to the ground, stopping when your elbows are at a 90° angle or your chest is 1–2 inches from the floor.   **3** Exhale and push up from the floor.   **4** As your arms near full extension, lift your left hand off the floor and slowly raise your hand up to the ceiling while simultaneously rotating your entire torso, head and left leg; your body should form a "T" shape with your left arm pointing directly upward and your right hand in contact with the floor, supporting your weight. Maintain a contracted core and keep your spine erect. Hold that position for 3 seconds (or longer if you choose to incorporate a side plank).   **5** Slowly rotate your torso back to plank position. Repeat on the other side.

PULL-UP

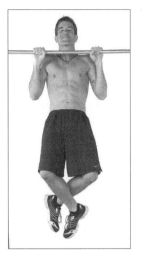

1 Grip the horizontal bar with your palms facing away from you and your arms fully extended. Your hands should be slightly wider (up to 2 inches) than your shoulders. Your feet should not touch the floor during this exercise. Let all of your weight settle in position but don't relax your shoulders—this may cause them to overstretch. **2** Squeeze your shoulder blades together to start the initial phase of the pull-up. During this initial movement, pretend that you're squeezing a pencil between your shoulder blades—don't let the pencil drop during any phase of the pull-up. For phase two, look up at the bar, exhale and pull your chin up toward the bar by driving your elbows toward your hips. It's very important to keep your shoulders back and chest up during the entire movement. Pull yourself up in a controlled manner until the bar is just above the top of your chest. **3** Inhale and lower yourself back to starting position.

ASSISTED PULL-UP: If you need a little assistance, you can set a stable chair behind you and place your toes on the seat, pushing up as needed to complete each rep. Another excellent option is to use an exercise band to get assistance while training with the full range of motion. Loop an exercise band over the bar and through, then place your knee in the bottom of the loop to provide some aid, primarily in the bottom portion of the exercise when your arms are at full extension. As you get stronger, progress to using less and less assistance.

CHIN-UP

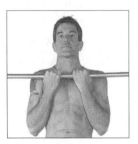

The Position Grab the bar with your palms facing you. This movement is easiest because it allows you to use more of your biceps to complete the motion. On average, underhand pull-ups are about 10–15 percent easier than overhand pull-ups.

ASSISTED CHIN-UP: See Assisted Pull-Ups above.

COMMANDO PULL-UP

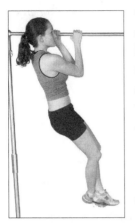

1 Stand perpendicular to the bar with it directly overhead and bisecting your body into left and right halves. Reach up to grip the bar like a baseball bat (e.g., hands on opposite sides of the bar). Your elbows should be a few inches apart and pointed toward the floor, not flared out to the sides. **2** Engage your core and pull upward using your biceps, shoulder, chest and back to bring your head up on one side of the bar. Keep your arms tight to your torso and bring your elbows toward your waist. At the top of the move, touch one shoulder to the bar. **3** In a slow and controlled manner, lower your body back to the starting position. Switch shoulders each rep.

ADVANCED VARIATION: For more core activation, on the upward movement raise your knees up and crunch your core—the higher your legs, the more you activate your core. You can even bring your feet up to touch the bar.

V-SIT

This is a slow, controlled movement: Never jerk your body from a prone dorsal position to a V—that's a quick way to pull a muscle! Really focus on your form and practice keeping your core engaged and mirroring the straightness of your upper body and legs. It also doesn't hurt to have a soft cushion under your tailbone.

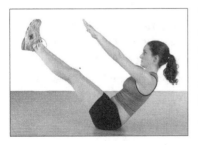

1 Lie flat on your back with your legs extended straight along the floor and your arms extended overhead on the floor with your biceps by your ears. **2** Contracting your abdominal muscles and keeping your legs straight, raise your legs and upper torso to form a "V." Your straight arms can be held parallel to your legs or alongside your ears. Hold the position for at least 3 seconds. **3** Slowly lower everything down without touching the ground with your heels or shoulders, then perform another rep.

REVERSE CRUNCH

Keep your back straight and lower legs on a level plane throughout this slow and controlled movement.

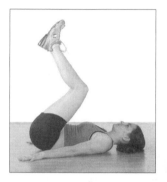

1 Lie flat on your back with your legs extended along the floor and your arms along your sides, palms down.   **2** Contracting your lower abdominal muscles, lift your feet 4–6 inches off the floor, bend your knees and bring them in toward your chest. Be careful not to put excessive pressure on your lower back by bringing your hips off the floor. Pause when your glutes rise slightly off the mat.   **3** Extend your legs and lower them until your feet are 4–6 inches off the floor.

HANGING LEG RAISE

This is a great movement to work your lower abdominal muscles and hips while also providing a great stretch for your arms, shoulders and back. Don't be surprised if your vertebrae re-align themselves when you first hang and even throughout the move.

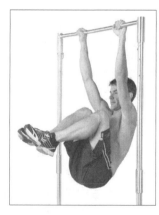

1 Grab an overhead bar with your preferred grip (underhand, overhand or mixed) and hang from the bar with your arms fully extended but elbows not locked. For this exercise, count 3 seconds up, hold 1–3 seconds, and then 3 seconds down.   **2** Contracting your abdominal muscles, slowly bring your knees up toward your chest while keeping your torso as close to vertical as possible. Don't lean back during the movement or swing between reps.   **3** Lower your legs in the same slow manner.

BICYCLE CRUNCH

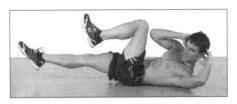

1 Lie flat on your back with your legs extended straight along the floor and your hands at both sides of your head, fingers touching your temples. **2** Raise your feet 6 inches off the floor while simultaneously contracting your rectus abdominis and lifting your upper back and shoulders off the floor. In one movement, bend your left knee and raise your left leg so that the thigh and shin are at 90º; rotate your torso using your oblique muscles so that your right elbow touches the inside of your left knee. **3** Rotate your torso back to center and lower your upper body toward the floor, stopping before your shoulders touch. **4** Extend your left knee and return your foot to 6 inches off the floor and bend your right leg to 90º. Contract your abs, rotate and touch your left elbow to the inside of your right knee. This is 2 reps.

SUPERMAN

Interestingly enough, this exercise is not performed "up, up and away" but actually on your stomach, flat on the ground. This move strengthens your lower back and gives some due attention to your erector spinae—you know, those muscles that keep you vertical.

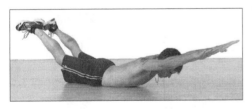

1 Lying face down on your stomach, extend your arms directly out in front of you and your legs behind you. Keep your knees straight as if you were flying. **2** In a slow and controlled manner, contract your erector spinae and raise your arms and legs about 6–8 inches off the floor. Hold for 5 seconds. **3** Lower slowly back to starting position.

SQUAT

Squat form is crucial to getting the most out of this extremely beneficial exercise. Check out your form by using a full-body mirror and standing perpendicular to it as you complete your reps.

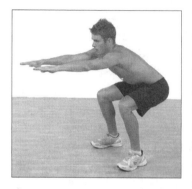

1 Stand tall with your feet shoulder-width apart and toes pointed slightly outward, about 11 and 1 o'clock. Raise your arms until they're parallel to the floor. **2** Bend at the hips and knees and "sit back" just a little bit as if you were about to sit directly down into a chair. Keep your head up, eyes forward and arms out in front of you for balance. As you descend, contract your glutes while your body leans forward slightly so that your shoulders are almost in line with your knees. Your knees should not extend past your toes and your weight should remain between the heel and the middle of your feet—do not roll up on the balls of your feet. Stop when your knees are at 90º and your thighs are parallel to the floor. If you feel your weight is on your toes or heels, adjust your posture and balance until your weight is in the middle of your feet. Squats should be a very stable movement—that is, until you try the one-legged variety! **3** Push straight up from your heels back to starting position. Don't lock your knees at the top of the exercise. This is 1 rep.

AIR SQUAT: For this version, lower yourself into a squat position then swing your arms up and explode straight up in the air. Land softly on your feet.

SQUAT WITH MEDICINE BALL

The medicine ball provides some additional weight to the squat and also works your arms, core and a litany of connecting muscles by changing your point of balance throughout the move. As an added benefit, it gives you something useful to do with your hands.

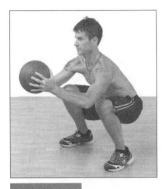

1 Stand tall with your feet shoulder-width apart and toes pointed slightly outward, about 11 and 1 o'clock. Hold a medicine ball at chest level.
2 Keeping the ball in front of you, perform a traditional squat. When your knees near 90º, stop and slowly return to standing. **3** Exhale and raise the ball straight up overhead.
4 Slowly lower the ball back to chest level.

LUNGE

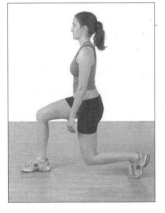

1 Stand tall with your feet shoulder-width apart and your arms hanging at your sides. **2** Take a large step forward with your right foot, bend both knees and drop your hips straight down until both knees are bent 90º. Your left knee should almost be touching the ground and your left toes are on the ground behind you. Keep your core engaged and your back, neck and hips straight at all times during this movement.
3 Pushing up with your right leg, straighten both knees and return to starting position. Repeat with the other leg.

LUNGE WITH TWIST

This movement is exactly like the forward or reverse lunge, but now your hands and core can get in on the fun.

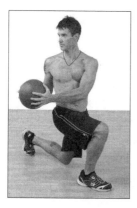

1 Stand tall with your feet shoulder-width apart and both hands on opposite sides of a medicine ball, elbows slightly bent. **2** Keeping the ball directly in front of you, step forward (or backward) with your right foot to start the lunge motion. As you lower your hips, twist your core and swing the ball laterally to your right until both knees are bent 90º and your arms are extended and holding the medicine ball to the right, 90º from where you started. **3** Return to starting position and repeat to the other side.

JUMPING LUNGES

1 Stand tall with your feet shoulder-width apart and your arms hanging at your sides. **2** Step backward with your left foot, bend both knees and drop your hips straight down until both knees are bent 90°. Your left knee should almost be touching the ground and your left toes are on the ground behind you. Keep your core engaged and your back, neck and hips straight at all times during this movement. Pushing up with your right leg, explosively straighten both knees and jump straight up in the air, switching your left and right leg position midair so you land with your right knee and toes behind you.

PLANK

This is a timed exercise, so place a watch where you can see it when you're in position.

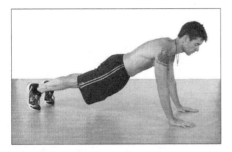

1 Place your hands on the ground approximately shoulder-width apart, making sure your fingers point straight ahead and your arms are straight but your elbows not locked. Step your feet back until your body forms a straight line from head to feet. Your feet should be about 6 inches apart with the weight in the balls of your feet. Engage your core to keep your spine from sagging; don't sink into your shoulders. Look at your watch and note the time—you're on the clock. **2** Lower to starting position when time is reached.

FOREARM PLANK

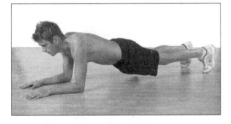

Place your elbows on the floor beneath your shoulders, your hands palm-down on the floor and your entire forearms in contact with the floor. Because your body is closer to parallel with the floor, you're working your core even harder to maintain a straight line from head to toe.

SIDE PLANK

The side plank is a great isolation exercise for tightening your internal and external abdominal obliques (aka your love handles) as well as the transverse abdominis. The instability of the side plank will work a host of supporting muscles all over your body, including your hips, glutes, chest and back. On average, side planks are held for about half as long as standard planks.

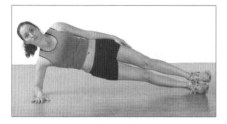

1 Lie on your side and stack your feet, hips and shoulders atop each other. Prop yourself up on your elbow, keeping it directly under your shoulder; your forearm should be completely on the ground, perpendicular to your body. **2** Engaging your core to keep your spine erect, lift your hips off the floor until you form a nice line from head to feet. Let your top arm rest along your side. Hold the position for a predetermined amount of time or for as long as possible. **3** Slowly lower your hips to the floor. Repeat on the opposite side.

IN & OUT

Aside from planks, this is my favorite core move due to its full range of motion and how well it works the entire rectus abdominis and erector spinae without putting excessive force on your upper spine and neck. This is a very slow and controlled motion and is performed best at a cadence of 3 seconds in, 3 seconds hold and 3 seconds out.

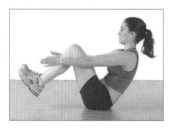

1 Lie flat on your back with your legs extended straight along the floor and your arms along your sides, palms down. **2** Lift your feet about 3 inches off the floor, bend your knees and bring your feet toward your butt while simultaneously lifting your arms off the floor and activating your abs to roll your upper body upward. **3** Continue raising your head and shoulders off the floor and bringing your hands past the outside of your knees while bringing your knees and chest together. At the top of the move, pause for 1-3 seconds. **4** Slowly return to starting position. Be careful to "roll" your spine in a natural movement and let your shoulders and head lightly touch the floor.

WOOD CHOP

For a somewhat easier version, this can also be done without a medicine ball.

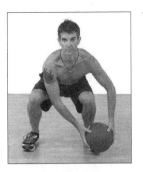

1 Stand tall with your feet shoulder-width apart, holding a medicine ball in front of you. **2** Lower your body into a squat until your knees are bent 90º, and bring the ball down to touch your left foot. **3** Stand tall, twisting your torso to the right and lifting your arms straight up over your head. Your left shoulder should be in front and you should be looking to the right. **4** Repeat to the other side.

MARCHING TWIST

Start slowly and work up the intensity. You can even throw in some intervals to really raise your heart rate.

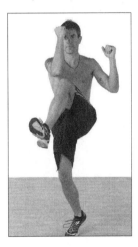

1 Stand tall with your feet shoulder-width apart. Bring your arms in front of you and bend your elbows 90º. **2** Twist your torso to the left and raise your left knee to your right elbow. **3** Repeat with your right knee and left elbow. A little hop with the bottom foot helps you keep your momentum going from leg to leg.

MASON TWIST

Always be careful when using weights in a twisting motion as you can easily injure your lower back. Start with the lightest possible weight and work your way up.

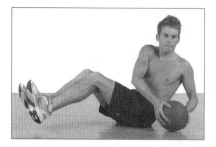

1 Sit on the floor with your knees comfortably bent, feet on the floor, arms bent 90° and hands holding a medicine ball or weight in front of your chest. **2** Lift your feet 4–6 inches off the floor and balance your bodyweight on your posterior. Keep your core tight to protect your back. **3** While maintaining the same hip position, twist your entire torso at the waist and touch the ball to the floor on the left side of your body. **4** Rotate back to center, keeping your feet off the floor and maintaining your balance using the supporting core muscles. Then rotate to your right and touch the ball to the floor. **5** Return to center. This is 1 rep.

> **MODIFICATION:** If you're not ready to add weight, you can also do this by clasping your hands in front of you.

MOUNTAIN CLIMBER

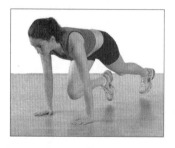

1 Assume the top position of a push-up with your hands directly under your shoulders and toes on the ground. Keep your core engaged and your body in a straight line from head to toe. **2** Lift your right toe slightly off the ground, bring your right knee to your chest and place your right foot on the ground under your body. **3** With a very small hop from both feet extend your right foot back to starting position and at the same time bring your left knee to your chest and place your left foot on the ground under your body. **4** Continue switching, making sure to keep your hips low.

JUMPING JACKS

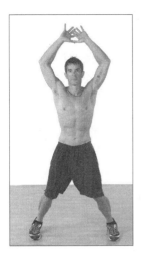

1 Stand tall with your feet together and arms extended along your sides, palms facing forward. **2** Jump 6–12 inches off the ground and simultaneously spread your feet apart an additional 20–30 inches while extending your hands directly overhead. **3** Jump 6–12 inches off the ground and return your hands and feet to starting position.

BURPEE

The burpee combines a squat, a double-leg mountain climber, a push-up and a high jump. It's a great full-body workout that you can do anywhere to work up a sweat and target your arms, chest, glutes, quads, hamstrings, calves and core. Since it's a multiple-position movement, take the time to learn and practice proper position for each move before you try it at full speed.

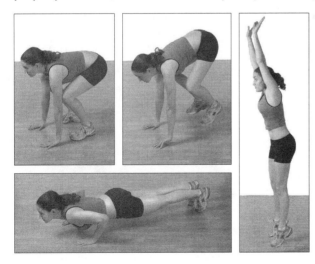

1 Stand tall with your back erect, feet shoulder-width apart and toes rotated slightly outward. **2** Shift your hips backward and "sit back" for the squat, keeping your head up and bending your knees. Lean your weight forward and place your hands on the floor, inside, outside or in front of your feet—whichever is more comfortable and gives you a nice, stable base.   **3** Kick your feet straight back so that you're now in a push-up starting position, forming a nice line from your head to your feet. Keep your core tight to maintain an erect spine.   **4** Inhale as you lower your torso toward the floor for a push-up. Stop when your body is 1–2 inches from the floor.   **5** Exhaling, straighten your arms and propel your entire upper body off the floor while simultaneously bending your knees and bringing them toward your chest in order to plant your feet underneath you. You should end up back in the bottom position of a squat. Take a quick breath.   **6** Swing your arms straight overhead, exhale and push off from your feet to jump straight up in the air as high as possible. Land with your knees slightly bent to absorb the impact. That's 1 rep.

FLUTTER KICK

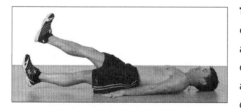

1 Lie flat on your back with your legs extended along the floor and your arms along your sides, palms down.   **2** Contract your lower abdominal muscles and lift your feet 6 inches off the floor. Hold for 5 seconds. (I prefer to flex my feet 90º in order to work my calves a bit, but you may point your toes.)   **3** While keeping your left foot in place, lift your right foot 6 inches higher (it should now be 12 inches off the floor). Hold for 5 seconds.   **4** Simultaneously lower your right leg back to 6 inches off the floor while raising your left foot 6 inches higher. Hold for 5 seconds. This counts as 2 reps.

BUTT KICK

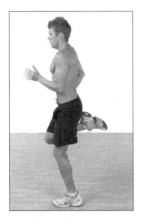

Run forward by taking very small steps and raising the heel of your back leg up toward your buttocks. Push forward from the ball of your grounded foot, progressing 12 to 18 inches per stride.

HIP RAISE

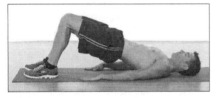

1 Lie on your back with your knees bent and feet flat on the floor, as close to your butt as possible. Extend your hands toward your hips and place your arms and palms flat on the floor at your sides. **2** Engage your abdominal muscles to keep your core tight, and exhale while you press your feet into the floor and raise your hips and lower back up, forming a straight line from your sternum to your knees. Do not push your hips too high or arch your back. Hold this position for 3–5 seconds. **3** Inhale and slowly return to starting position. That's 1 rep.

HIGH KNEES

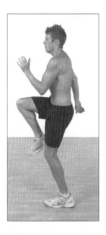

Run forward using a normal-length stride. Bend the knee of your elevated leg 90° and raise it until it's level with your waist. Push forward from the ball of your grounded foot, switch legs, and repeat. Pump your arms to generate leg drive and speed.

INCHWORM

This is a great full-body exercise and a perfect test for hamstring and lower back flexibility. In this motion-based exercise, you'll advance forward approximately 4 feet per repetition, so plan your exercise positioning accordingly.

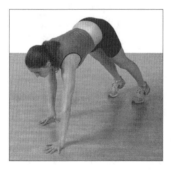

1 Stand with your feet about hip-width apart and fold over so that your hands touch the floor. **2** Keeping your hands firmly on the floor to balance your weight, walk your hands out in front of you one at a time until you're at the top of a push-up. Hold for 3 seconds. **3** Keeping your hands firmly on the floor to balance your weight, "walk" your feet toward your head by taking very small steps on your toes. Imagine that your lower legs are bound together and you can only bend your feet at each ankle. As you continue walking your feet toward your head, your butt will rise and your body will form an inverse "V." When you've stretched your hamstrings, glutes and calves as far as you can, hold that position for 3 seconds. That's 1 rep.

WARM-UPS & STRETCHES

Since you'll be pushing, pressing and lifting your bodyweight, it's very important to warm up before you stretch. Stretching prior to warming up can cause more damage than good to muscles, ligaments and joints. When your muscles are cold, they're far less pliable and you don't receive any benefit from stretching prior to warming up. Below are some dynamic warm-ups that'll get your heart rate up, loosen tight muscles and prepare you for your workout.

After your workout, stretching will help you reduce soreness, increase range of motion and flexibility within a joint or muscle, and prepare your body for any future workouts. Stretching immediately post-exercise while your muscles are still warm allows your muscles to return to their full range of motion (which gives you more flexibility gains) and reduces the chance of injury or fatigue in the hours or days after an intense workout.

It's important to remember that even when you're warm and loose, you should never "bounce" during stretching. Keep your movements slow and controlled. The stretches in this section should be performed in order to optimize your recovery. Remember to exhale as you perform every deep stretch and rest 30 seconds in between each stretch.

ARM CIRCLE

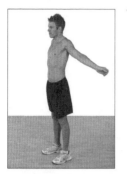

1 Stand with your feet shoulder-width apart. **2** Move both arms in a complete circle forward 5 times and then backward 5 times.

LUMBER JACK

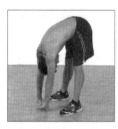

1 Stand with your feet shoulder-width apart and extend your hands overhead with elbows locked, fingers interlocked, and palms up. **2** Bend forward at the waist and try to put your hands on the ground (like you're chopping wood). **3** Raise up and repeat.

SIDE BEND

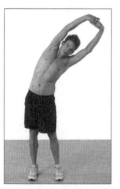

1 Stand with your feet shoulder-width apart and extend your hands overhead with elbows locked, fingers interlocked and palms up. **2** Bend side to side.

AROUND THE WORLD

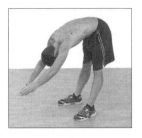

1 Stand with your feet shoulder-width apart and extend your hands overhead with elbows locked, fingers interlocked, and palms up. Keep your arms straight the entire time. **2** Bending at the hips, bring your hands down toward your right leg, and in a continuous circular motion bring your hands toward your toes, then toward your left leg and then return your hands overhead and bend backward. **3** Repeat three times, then change directions.

BARN DOOR

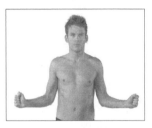

1 Stand with your feet shoulder-width apart with your arms tight against your sides. Bend your arms 90º so that your forearms extend forward and are parallel to the floor. Grip your hands like you have a rubber band between them. **2** Keeping your forearms parallel to the floor, squeeze your shoulder blades together and pull your hands apart to the sides. Do 10–12 repetitions.

CHEST FLY

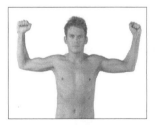

1 Assume the Barn Doors position (above) with your hands in front of your torso, then raise your hands and elbows straight up, maintaining the 90º angle until your elbows are at shoulder height. **2** Squeezing your shoulder blades together, pull your hands away from each other until your hands are parallel to your ears. Do 10–12 repetitions.

INDEX